MW00467120

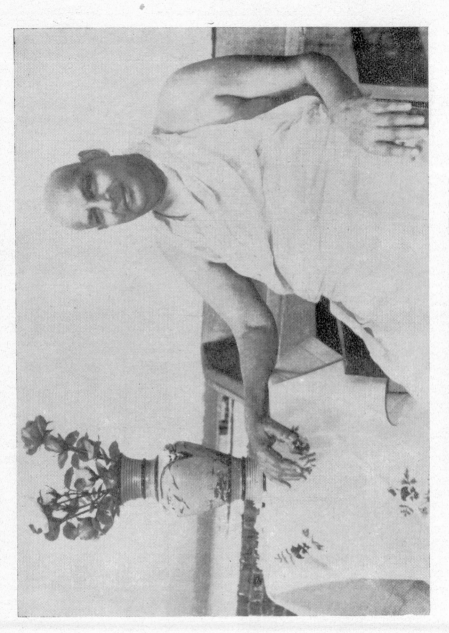

H.H. SRI SWAMI SIVANANDAJI MAHARAJ

DHYANA YOGA

Swami Sivananda

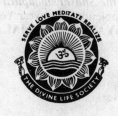

Published By
THE DIVINE LIFE SOCIETY
P.O. SHIVANANDANAGAR—249 192
Distt. Tehri-Garhwal, U.P., Himalayas, India

Price]   1994   [Rs. 40/-

Sixth Edition: 1994
(4,000 Copies)

© The Divine Life Trust Society

Printed on the happy occasion
of the Shashtyabdapurti
(completion of 60 years) of
SRI VIJAYARATNAM, MALAYSIA
(1000 Copies)

ISBN 81-7052-036-3

Published by Swami Krishnananda
for The Divine Life Society, Shivanandanagar, and
printed by him at the Yoga-Vedanta Forest Academy Press,
P.O. Shivanandanagar, Distt. Tehri-Garhwal,
U.P., Himalayas, India

PUBLISHERS' NOTE

Meditation is the key which unlocks the treasure-trove of the highest intelligence, of wisdom, of divinity, of genius. No man who wishes to make a success of his life can afford to neglect it.

The genius among scientists, the successful businessman, the best among philosophers, the Yogi and the seeker after Truth, all of them meditate. Their achievements are the fruits of their meditation.

The secrets of meditation have remained the close preserve of Yogis, till the Sage of the Himalayas, Sri Swami Sivanandaji Maharaj, in his supreme compassion and all-consuming love for all mankind, came forward to elucidate the philosophical foundation, the method, the experiences, the obstacles and the successful fulfilment of meditation.

His writings on this vital subject are presented by him in this inspiring book.

THE DIVINE LIFE SOCIETY

iii

PREFACE

Dhyana or meditation is in the keeping up of the flow of one idea with a continuity as unbroken as the flow of oil. Meditation is of two kinds, viz., concrete and abstract. If you meditate on any picture or concrete object it is concrete meditation. If you meditate on an abstract idea, on any quality such as mercy, tolerance, it is abstract meditation. A beginner should practise concrete meditation. For some aspirants, abstract meditation is more easy than concrete meditation.

The practice of meditation must start only after one is well established in Pratyahara or abstraction of the senses and concentration. If the senses are turbulent, if the mind cannot be fixed on one point, no meditation is possible even within hundreds of years. One should go stage by stage, step by step. The mind should be withdrawn again and again and fixed upon the object of meditation. Its tendency to run and roam must be checked. One should reduce one's wants and renounce all sorts of wild, vain desires from the mind. A desireless man alone can sit quiet and practise meditation. Sattvic and light diet and Brahmacharya are the prerequisites for the practice of meditation.

Consciousness is of two kinds, viz., focussing consciousness and marginal consciousness. When you concentrate on Trikuti, the space midway between the eyebrows, your focussing consciousness is on the Trikuti. When some flies sit on your left hand during meditation, you drive them with your right hand. When you become conscious of the flies it is called marginal consciousness. A seed which has remained in the fire for a second will not undoubtedly sprout into leaves even though sown in a fertile soil. Even so a mind that does meditation for some time but runs towards sensual objects on account of unsteadiness will not bring in the full fruits of Yoga.

Beginners on the spiritual path should remember again and again some important and inspiring Vedantic statements, every day. Only then can their doubts be removed and they would find themselves established on the path. Some of these statements are: "Being alone was in the beginning, one without a second" Chhandogya Upanishad Vl-2-1; "In the beginning all this was the one Self alone" Aitareya Upanishad VI-2-1; "This is the Brahman, without cause and without effect; this Self is Brahman perceiving everything" Brihadaranyaka Upanishad II-5-19; "That immortal Brahman alone is" Mandukya Upanishad, II-2-7. This immortal Atman cannot be attained without constant practice of meditation. Therefore he who wishes to attain immortality and freedom should meditate on the Self or the Brahman, for a long time.

The Self or the Atman is the fountain-source of all energy. Thinking on Atman as the Source of all Energy, is a dynamic method for augmenting one's own energy, strength and power. If you think even for a single second, of the all-pervading pure, immortal Satchidananda Atman or Brahman, it would be tantamount to taking thousand and eight dips in the sacred Triveni—the junction of holy rivers at Prayag. This is the real mental sacred bath. Physical bath is nothing when compared to this internal bath of wisdom or knowledge.

Worship the Self or the Atman with the flowers of Jnana or wisdom, contentment, peace, joy and equal vision. This will constitute real worship. Offerings of rose, jasmine, sandal paste, incense, sweetmeats and fruits are nothing when compared to the offerings of Jnana, contentment, peace, equal vision. These are the offerings given by the ignorant persons. Try to identify yourself with the eternal, immortal, ever-pure Atman or Soul that resides in the chambers of your heart. Think and feel always: "I am the very pure Atman. This one thought will remove all troubles and fanciful thoughts. The mind wants to delude you when it detracts you from the central purpose of your life, viz., meditation on the Atman. Therefore start an anti-current of thought against the tendencies of the mind. Then, mind will lurk like a thief and become submissive.

In the Yoga-Vasishtha you will find: "The right course to be adopted by one who is a novitiate is this: Two parts of the mind must be filled with the objects of enjoyments, one part with philosophy and the remaining part with devotion to the teacher. Having advanced a little, he should fill one part of the mind with the object of enjoyment, two parts with devotion to the teacher and the remaining one with getting an insight into the meaning of philosophy. When one has attained proficiency, he should every day fill two parts of his mind with philosophy and supreme Renunciation, and the remaining two parts with meditation and devoted service to the Guru." This will eventually lead you on to meditation for twenty-four hours. Meditate ceaselessly upon that Satchidananda Brahman and attain the Supreme immaculate seat in this very life.

INTRODUCTION

1. The Science of Meditation

Concentration is holding the mind on to some particular object. An unbroken flow of knowledge in that subject is meditation. Meditation is regular flow of thought with regard to the object of concentration. Meditation follows concentration. Concentration merges in meditation. Meditation opens the doors of the mind to intuitive knowledge and many powers. You can get whatever you want through meditation. During meditation all worldly thoughts are shut out from the mind. Meditation is called Dhyana in Sanskrit and is the seventh step in the Yogic Ladder.

There should be a separate room for meditation and other spiritual exercises and practices. The room should be regarded as a temple of God. You should not allow anybody into the room. You should enter the room with a pious and reverent mind. Thoughts of jealousy, lust, greed and anger should not be entertained within the four walls of the room. All worldly talks also should not be indulged in there. For every word that is uttered, every thought that is cherished and every deed that is done is not lost; they are reflected on the subtle layers of ether encircling the room where they are done and hence affect the mind, invariably.

Decorate the room with inspiring pictures of great Saints, Sages, Prophets and World Teachers. In a prominent place in the room keep a beautiful photo of your tutelary Deity (Ishta-Devata), either Lord Jesus, Lord Krishna, Lord Siva or Devi. Let the Deity face the East or North. Spread your Asana

vii

(seat) in front of the Deity. Keep some religious and philosophical books such as the Bhagavad-Gita, the Upanishads, the Vedanta-Sutras, the Ramayana, the Yogavasishtha, the Bible, etc., by your side. Wash your face, hands and legs before you enter the room. Burn a piece of camphor and light some scented sticks immediately after entering the room. Sit on the Asana in front of the Deity and repeat the Name of the Lord or sing some devotional hymns. Then take to the practice of concentration and meditation.

We cannot seek for ideal places. Even if we wander from pole to pole, we cannot get an ideal place that will satisfy us from every standpoint. Every place has some advantages and some disadvantages as well. So you should select a place that is more advantageous than the others. Having once selected a place, you must stick to it till the last. You must not think of changing the place, when some difficulty stares you in the face. You must put up with the difficulty by all means. Rishikesh (Himalayas), Hardwar, Uttarkashi, Badrinarayan, Gangotri, Mount Kailas, Brindawan, Banaras, Nasik and Ayodhya are all excellent places for meditation in India.

The best and the most congenial time for the practice of meditation is unquestionably the Brahmamuhurta, i.e., from 4 to 6 a.m. That is the time when the mind is quite refreshed after an agreeable slumber, when the mind is calm and comparatively pure. It is like a clean blank sheet of paper. Only such a mind can be moulded into whatever shape you like. Moreover, the atmosphere also is charged with purity and goodness at this time.

In the beginning you can meditate twice daily, from 4 to 5 in the morning and 7 to 8 at night. As you advance in your practices you can increase the duration of each sitting little by little using your commonsense and discretion, and also have a third sitting either in the morning between 10 and 11 or in the evening between 4 and 5.

Sitting on your favourite meditative pose and keeping the head, neck and trunk erect, close your eyes and gently

viii

concentrate on either the tip of the nose, space between the eyebrows, the heart-lotus or the crown of the head. When once you have selected one centre of concentration, stick to it till the last with leechlike tenacity. Never change it. Thus, if you have chosen to concentrate on the heart-lotus after having tried the other centres, stick to the heart-lotus alone. Then only can you expect rapid advancement.

Meditation is of two kinds, viz., Saguna (with Gunas or qualities) meditation and Nirguna (without Gunas or qualities) meditation. Meditation on Lord Krishna, Lord Siva, Lord Rama or Lord Jesus is Saguna meditation. It is meditation with form and attributes. The Name of the Lord is also simultaneously repeated. This is the method of the Bhaktas. Meditation on the reality of the Self is Nirguna meditation. This is the method of the Vedantins. Meditation on Om, Soham, Sivoham, Aham Brahma Asmi and Tat Twam Asi is Nirguna meditation.

Put an iron rod in the blazing furnace. It becomes red like fire. Remove it from the fire. It loses its red colour. If you want to keep it always red, you must keep it always in fire. Even so, if you want to keep the mind charged with the fire of Brahmic Wisdom, you must keep it always in contact with the Brahmic Fire of Knowledge through constant and intense meditation. You must, in other words, keep up an unceasing flow of Brahmic consciousness.

Meditation is the most powerful mental and nervine tonic. The holy vibrations penetrate all the cells of the body and cure the various diseases that human flesh is heir to. Those who regularly meditate save the doctor's bills. The powerful soothing waves that arise during meditation exercise a benign influence on the mind, nerves, organs and cells of the body. The divine energy freely flows like the flow of oil from one vessel to another, from the Feet of the Lord to the different systems of the practitioner.

If you meditate for half an hour, you will be able to face the daily battle of life with peace and spiritual strength for one week through the force of meditation. Such is the beneficial effect of meditation. As you have to move with different minds of peculiar nature, get the requisite strength and peace from meditation and be free from worry and trouble.

The wise cut asunder the knot of egoism by the sharp sword of constant meditation. Then draw supreme Knowledge of the Self or full illumination or Self-realisation. All bonds of Karma (action) are rent asunder. Therefore be ever engaged in meditation. This is the master-key to open the realms of eternal Bliss. It may be disgusting and tiring in the beginning, because the mind will be running away from the point (Lakshya) every now and then. But after sometime it will be focussed in the centre. You will be immersed in Divine Bliss.

Regular meditation opens up the avenues of intuitional knowledge, makes the mind calm and steady, awakens an ecstatic feeling, and brings the Yogic student in contact with the Supreme Purusha. If there are doubts, they are all cleared by themselves, when you march on the path of Dhyana-Yoga (meditation) steadily. You will yourself feel the way to place your footstep in the next higher rung of the Yogic ladder. A mysterious inner voice will guide you. Hear thou this attentively, O Aspirant!

When you get a flash of illumination, do not be frightened. It will be a new experience of immense joy. Do not turn back. Do not give up meditation. Do not stop there. You will have to advance still further. This is only a glimpse of truth. This is not the highest realisation. This is only a new platform. Try to ascend further. Reach the Bhuma or the Infinite. Now alone you are proof against all temptations. You will drink deep the nectar of Immortality. This is the acme or final stage. You will take eternal rest now. You need not meditate any further. This is the final goal.

You have within yourself tremendous powers and latent faculties of which you have really never had any conception. You must awaken these dormant powers and faculties by the practice of meditation and Yoga. You must develop your will and control your senses and mind. You must purify yourself and practise regular meditation. Then only can you become a Superman or God-man.

There is no such thing as miracle or Siddhi. Ordinary man is quite ignorant of higher spiritual things. He is sunk in oblivion. He is shut up from higher transcendental knowledge. So he calls some extraordinary event a miracle. But for a Yogi who understands things in the light of Yoga, there is no such thing as miracle. Just as a villager is astonished at the sight of an aeroplane or a talkie for the first time, so also a man of the world is stunned when he sees an extraordinary spectacle for the first time.

Every human being has within himself various potentialities and capacities. He is a magazine of power and knowledge. As he evolves, he unfolds new powers, new faculties, new qualities. Now he can change his environments and influence others. He can subdue other minds. He can conquer internal and external nature. He can enter into superconscious state.

In a dark room if a pot containing a lamp inside it is broken, the darkness of the room is dispelled and you see light everywhere in the room. Even so, if the body-pot is broken through constant meditation on the Self, i.e., if you destroy ignorance (Avidya) and its effects such as identification with the body, and rise above body-consciousness you will cognise the supreme light of the Atman everywhere.

Just as the water in the pot that is placed in the ocean becomes one with the waters of the ocean, when the pot is broken, so also when the body-pot is broken by meditation on the Atman, the individual soul becomes one with the Supreme Soul.

Just as the light is burning within the hurricane lamp, so also the Divine Flame is burning from the time immemorial in the lamp of your heart. Close your eyes. Merge yourself within the Divine Flame. Plunge deep into the chambers of your heart. Meditate on this Divine Flame and become one with the Flame of God.

If the wick within the lamp is small, the light will also be small. If the wick is big, the light also will be powerful. Similarly if the Jiva (individual soul) is pure, if he practises meditation, the manifestation or expression of the Self will be powerful. He will radiate a big light. If he is unregenerate and impure, he will be like a burnt-up charcoal. The bigger the wick, the greater the light. Likewise, the purer the soul, the greater the expression.

If the magnet is powerful, it will influence the iron filings even when they are placed at a distance. Even so, if the Yogi is an advanced person, he will have greater influence over the persons with whom he comes in contact. He can exert his influence on persons even when they live in distant places.

The fire of meditation annihilates all foulness due to vice. Then suddenly there comes Knowledge of the Self or Divine Wisdom which directly leads to Mukti or final emancipation.

During the meditation note how long you can shut out all worldly thoughts. Watch your mind. If it is for twenty minutes, try to increase the period to thirty minutes and so on. Fill the mind with thoughts of God again and again.

In meditation do not strain your eyes. Do not struggle or wrestle with the mind. Relax. Gently allow the divine thoughts to flow. Steadily think of the Lakshya (point of meditation). Do not voluntarily and violently drive away the intruding thoughts. Have sublime Sattvic thoughts. The vicious thoughts will by themselves vanish.

If there is much strain in your meditation, reduce the duration of each sitting for a few days. Do light meditation only. When you have regained the normal tone, again increase the period. Use your commonsense throughout your Sadhana. I always reiterate on this point.

"Though men perform Tapas standing on one leg, for a period of 1,000 years, it will not, in the least, be equal to one-sixteenth part of Dhyana-Yoga (meditation)." **Paingala Upanishad.**

Those who meditate for four or five hours at a stretch can have two meditative poses. Sometimes the blood accumulates in one part of the legs or thighs and so gives a little trouble. After two hours change the pose. Or stretch the legs at full length and lean against a wall or pillow. Keep the spine erect. This is the most comfortable Asana. Or join two chairs. Sit in one chair and stretch the legs on another chair. This is another contrivance.

You must daily increase your Vairagya, meditation and Sattvic virtues such as patience, perseverance, mercy, love, forgiveness, etc. Vairagya and good qualities help meditation. Meditation increases the Sattvic qualities.

Considerable changes take place in the mind, brain and nervous system by the practice of meditation. New nerve-currents, new vibrations, new avenues, new grooves, new cells, new channels are formed. The whole mind and the nervous system are remodelled. You will have a new heart, a new mind, new sensations; new feelings, new mode of thinking and acting and a new view of the universe (as God in manifestation).

During meditation you will get into rapture or ecstasy. It is of five kinds, viz., the lesser thrill, momentary rapture, flooding rapture, transporting rapture and all-pervading rapture. The lesser thrill will raise the hairs of the body (like the goose skin). The momentary rapture is like the productions of lightning moment by moment. Like waves breaking on the sea-shore, the flooding rapture descends rapidly on the body and breaks. Transporting rapture is strong and lifts the body up to the extent of launching it into the air. When the all-pervading rapture arises, the whole body is completely surcharged and blown like a full bladder.

"Whatever he (the Yogic practitioner) sees with his eyes, let him consider as Atman. Whatever he hears with his ears, let him consider as Atman. Whatever he smells with his nose, let him consider as Atman. Whatever he tastes with his tongue, let him consider as Atman. Whatever the Yogi touches with his skin, let him consider as Atman. The Yogi should thus unweariedly gratify his organs of sense for a period of one Yama (3 hours) every day with great effort. The various wonderful powers are attained by the Yogi, such as clairvoyance, clairaudience, ability to transport himself to great distances within a moment, great powers of speech, ability to take any form, ability to become invisible and the transmutation of iron into gold, when the former is smeared over with his excretion." **Yogatattva Upanishad.**

Just as a very skilful archer in shooting at a bird is aware of the way in which he takes his steps, holds the bow-string, and the arrow at the time when he pierces the bird, thus "standing in this position, holding thus the bow, thus the bow-string, and thus the arrow, I pierce the bird," and ever afterwards would not fail to fulfil these conditions that he might pierce the bird, even so the aspirant should note the conditions such as suitable food, thus "eating this kind of food, following such a person, in such a dwelling, in this mode, at this time, I attained, to this meditation and Samadhi."

As a clever cook in serving his master notes the kind of food that his master relishes and thenceforward serves it and gets gain, so the aspirant too notes the conditions such as nourishment, etc., at the moment of attaining meditation and Samadhi and in fulfilling them gets ecstasy again and again.

Leading a virtuous life is not by itself sufficient for God-realisation. Concentration of mind is absolutely necessary. A good virtuous life only prepares the mind as a fit instrument for concentration and meditation. It is concentration and meditation that eventually lead to Self-realisation or God-realisation.

"A Yogi should always avoid fear, anger, laziness, too much sleep or waking and too much food and fasting. If the above rules be well strictly practised each day, spiritual wisdom will arise of itself in three months without doubt. In four months, he sees the Devas; in five months, he knows (or becomes) Brahmanishtha; and truly in six months, he attains Kaivalya at will. There is no doubt." **Amritananda-Upanishad.**

During meditation some of the visions that you see are your own materialised thoughts, while some others are real objective visions. In meditation new grooves are formed in the brain and the mind moves upwards in the new spiritual grooves. In meditation and concentration you will have to train the mind in a variety of ways. Then only the gross mind will become subtle.

When you first practise meditation, lights of various colours such as red, white, blue, green, and a mixture of red and green, etc., will appear in the forehead. These are Tanmatric (elemental) lights. Every element has got its own colour. Water has white colour. Fire has red colour. Air has green colour. Ether has blue colour. So the coloured lights are due to these Tattvas (elements) only.

Sometimes you may see a big blazing sun or moon or lightning in front of the forehead. Do not mind these. Shun them. Try to dive deep into the source of these lights.

Sometimes Devatas, Nitya Siddhas (eternally perfected Yogis) and Amarapurushas (immortal beings) will appear in meditation. Receive them all with due honour. Bow down before them. Get advice from them. Do not be frightened. They appear before you to give you all spiritual help and encouragement.

"Having made Atman as the lower Arani (sacrificial wood) and the Pranava as the upper Arani, one should see God in secret through the practice of churning which is Dhyana (meditation)." **Dhyanabindu Upanishad.**

EXERCISES

I

Place a picture of Lord Jesus in front of you. Sit in your favourite meditative pose. Concentrate gently with open eyes on the picture till tears trickle down your cheeks. Rotate the mind on the cross, on the chest, long hairs, beautiful beard, round eyes, and the various other limbs of his body; and the fine spiritual aura emanating from his head, and so on. Think of the divine attributes such as love, magnanimity, mercy and forbearance. Think of the various phases of his interesting life and the 'miracles' he performed and the various 'extraordinary' powers he possessed. Then close your eyes and try to visualise the picture. Repeat the same process again and again.

II

Place a picture of Lord Hari in front of you. Sit again in your meditative posture. Concentrate gently on the picture till you shed tears. Rotate the mind on His feet, legs, yellow silken robes, golden garland set with diamonds, Koustubha gem, etc., on the chest, the earrings, then the face, the crown of the head, the discus on the right upper hand, the conch on the left upper hand, the mace on the right lower hand, and the lotus flower on the left lower hand. Then close the eyes and try to visualise the picture. Repeat the same process again and again.

III

Keep a picture of Lord Krishna with flute in hands in front of you. Sit in your meditative pose and gently concentrate on the picture till you shed tears. Think of his feet adorned with anklets, yellow garment, various ornaments

xvi

round His neck, the necklace set with the Koustubha gem, the long garland of beautiful flowers of various colours, earrings, crown set with precious jewels of priceless value, dark and long hairs, sparkling eyes, the *tilaka* in the forehead, the magnetic aura round His head, long hands adorned with bracelets and armlets, and the flute in the hands ready to be played upon. Then close your eyes and visualise the picture. Repeat the same process again and again.

IV

This is one kind of meditation for beginners. Sit on Padmasana in your meditation room. Close your eyes. Meditate on the effulgence in the sun, or the splendour in the moon or the glory in the stars.

V

Meditate on the magnanimity of the ocean and its infinite nature. Then compare the ocean to the infinite Brahman, and the waves, foams and icebergs to the various names and forms. Identify yourself with the ocean. Become silent. Expand. Expand.

VI

This is another kind of meditation. Meditate on the Himalayas. Imagine that the Ganges takes its origin in the icy regions of Gangotri near Uttarakasi flows through Rishikesh, Hardwar, Benaras, and then enters into the Bay of Bengal near Gangasagar. Himalayas, Ganges and the Sea—these three thoughts only should occupy your mind. First take your mind to the icy regions of Gangotri, then along the Ganges and finally to the Sea. Rotate the mind in this manner for ten minutes.

VII

There is a living Universal Power that underlies all these names and forms. Meditate on this Power which is formless. This will terminate in the realisation of the Absolute, Nirguna, Nirakara (formless) Consciousness eventually.

xvii

VIII

Sit on Padmasana. Close your eyes. Gaze steadily on the formless air only. Concentrate on the air. Meditate on the all-pervading nature of the air. This will lead to the realisation of the nameless and formless Brahman, the One Living Truth.

IX

Sit on your meditative pose. Close your eyes. Imagine that there is a supreme, infinite effulgence hidden behind all these names and forms which is tantamount to the effulgence of crores of suns put together. This is another form of Nirguna meditation.

X

Concentrate and meditate on the expansive blue sky. This is another kind of Nirguna meditation. By the previous methods of concentration the mind will cease thinking of finite forms. It will slowly begin to melt in the ocean of Peace, as it is deprived of its contents. The mind will become subtler and subtler.

XI

Have the picture of OM in front of you. Concentrate gently on this picture with open eyes till tears flow profusely. Associate the ideas of eternity, infinity, immortality, etc., when you think of OM. The humming of bees, the sweet notes of the nightingale, the seven tunes in music and all sounds are emanations from OM only. OM is the essence of the Vedas. Imagine that OM is the bow, the mind is the arrow and Brahman (God) is the target. Aim at the target with great care and then, like arrow becomes one with the target, you will become one with Brahman. The short accent of OM burns all sins, the long accent bestows all psychic powers (Siddhis). He who chants and meditates upon this monosyllable OM chants and meditates upon all the Scriptures of the world.

XII

Sit on Padmasana or Siddhasana in your meditation room. Watch the flow of breath. You will hear the sound.

"SOHAM", SO during inhalation and HAM during exhalation. SOHAM means I AM HE. The breath is reminding you of your identity with the Supreme Soul. You are unconsciously repeating Soham 21,600 times daily at the rate of 15 Sohams per minute. Associate the ideas of Existence, Knowledge, Bliss,. Absolute, Purity, Peace, Perfection, Love, etc., along with Soham. Negate the body while repeating the Mantra and identify yourself with the Atman or the Supreme Soul.

XIII

Uddhava asked Lord Krishna: "O Lotus-eyed ! How to meditate on Thee! Tell me what is the nature of that meditation and what it is?" To which Lord Krishna replied: "Be seated on the Asana that is neither high nor low, with your hands on the lap. Fix your gaze on the tip of the nose (in order to fix the mind). Purify the tracks of Prana by Puraka, Kumbhaka and Rechaka, and then again in the reverse way (i.e. first breathe in by the left nostril with the right nostril closed by the tip of the thumb, then close the nostril by the tips of the ring finger and the little finger and retain the breath in both the nostrils. Then remove the tip of the thumb and breathe out through the right nostril. Reverse the process by breathing in through the right nostril, then retaining the breath through the left nostril. Practise this Pranayama gradually with your senses controlled."

'Aum' with the sound of bell, extends all over, from Muladhara upwards. Raise the 'Aum' in the heart by means of Prana (twelve fingers upwards) as if it were the thread of a lotus-stalk. There let Bindu (the fifteenth vowel sound) be added to it. Thus practise Pranayama accompanied by the Pranava reciting the latter ten times. Continue the practice, three times a day, and within a month you shall be able to control the vital air. The lotus of the heart has its stalk upwards and the flower downwards facing below (and it is also closed, like the inflorescence with bracts of the banana). Meditate on it, however, as facing upwards and full-blown, with eight petals and with the pericarp. On the pericarp, think of the sun, the moon, and fire one after another. First meditate on all the limbs. Then let the mind withdraw the senses from their objects. Then draw the concentrated mind completely towards Me, by means of Buddhi (intellect). Then give up all other limbs and concentrate on one thing only, My smiling face. Do not meditate on any thing else. Then withdraw the concentrated mind from that and fix it on the Akasa (ether). Give up that also and being fixed in Me (as Brahman) think of nothing at all. You shall see Me in Atman, as identical with all Atmas."

CONTENTS

DHYANA YOGA

Chapter One

DHYANA YOGA EXPLAINED

1. MEDITATION—YOUR ONLY DUTY

Meditation is your only duty. You must realise the goal of your life: God-Realisation. Then only would your life be fruitful. There are several stages in the path to God-Realisation. Purification, concentration, reflection, meditation, illumination, identification, absorption and salvation. Through service you should purify yourself and then proceed through concentration, meditation, etc.; finally you reach the goal of Salvation.

Time for Meditation

You must do Brahma Vichara in Brahmamuhurtha. You must enquire "Who am I" in Brahmamuhurtha. Meditation performed for an hour in Brahmamuhurtha is equal to meditation performed for six hours during other periods of the day.

If you get up at 4 a.m. you will have time in the early morning for your prayers and meditation. You will charge yourself with Sattva. You will get strength to face the daily battle of life. Morning time is most suitable for meditation. The mind then is not filled with Raga-Dvesha as at other times. You can fill it with Sattva, through meditation, by recitation of Stotras and hymns, or of Slokas like "Ajo Nitya Sasvatoyam Puraano Na Hanyate Hanyamaane Shareere." You must ever dwell on these thoughts.

It is only for beginners: the instruction to meditate a little. You must meditate much. But you must increase the period gradually. Particularly retired people should meditate more. But, if I at once say, 'Meditate more', beginners will

be frightened. Therefore, I say 'Meditate a little' This is only
to tempt people to meditate first of all.

Method of Meditation

The mind is duping you every moment. Therefore, wake
up now at least and cultivate this discrimination through
enquiry into the nature of the Self, through Satsanga, study
and meditation.

Meditate on OM. 'Tad Japastadarthabhavanam'. OM is
Satchidananda. OM is infinity. Om is perfection and freedom.
Meditate on these divine attributes of Nirguna Brahman.

Meditate on the nature of the Self. 'I am Satchidananda—Existence-Knowledge-Bliss Absolute'. Meditate
on divine qualities. If you are not able to practise this abstract
meditation, then meditate on the Sun, the light, or the
all-pervading ether or air. Meditate on the light that is shining
in your heart; meditate on those dream pictures that you
sometimes get. Meditate on the form of your Guru or Saints.
Meditate on anything your mind likes best. Meditate on the
form of your father, on his qualities.

Do common meditation for a few minutes. From that
common meditation, you will know that real peace and bliss
are within. Collect all the rays of your mind—*Pratyagat-
manam Ishat Avrita Chakshuh*—repeat your Ishta Mantra: the
mind should not move towards the sense-objects, there is no
Vritti: Therefore, you enjoy perfect peace and bliss.
Regularly practise such meditation.

Nama Rupam Na Te Na Me

Aham Atma Nirakara Sarvavyapi Svabhavata.

Again and again meditate on these formulae. They will
give you strength. Even if you meditate once, it gives you
some strength.

You are not the body composed of the five elements.
Again and again remember this. Meditate on this. You must
find the Atman through reflection and meditation. "Atman

knows everything else; and knows itself, too." That is your real Svaroopa. There is no such object in this world.

Meditate and sing: 'Sivoham Sivoham Sivoham Soham. Satchidananda Svaroopoham.'

Practise Yoga Asanas and Pranayamas, which will purify the body and mind, remove all diseases and help in concentration and meditation.

You should get up in Brahmamuhurta and meditate. This is the best time for divine contemplation. The mind is calm. It is like a blank sheet of paper. You can mould it in any way you like. The worldly currents of Raga-Dvesha have not entered it at this time.

You can chant Om (long or Deergha Pranava) 10 or 12 times. When you so repeat Om all the Koshas will begin to vibrate harmoniously.

Meditate intensely, ceaselessly. It will be difficult to meditate ceaselessly in the beginning. Practise. You will grow in cheerfulness and joy. Increase the period of meditation. Gradually you will come to meditate ceaselessly, intensely.

Meditate on the abstract qualities like Existence. Knowledge and Bliss Absolute. Keep these thoughts always before your mind. This is the abstract background of thoughts. Or, you can meditate on the form of the Lord: Saguna Upasana. Mentally visualise the picture of the Lord. Now look at His Face, now at His Chakra, now at His Feet. The mind will not run.

The mind must not run out. If you try to find the mind on the Lord dwelling in the chambers of your heart you will be an introvert.

You can meditate on the Jyotis in the heart. You can meditate on the divine objects seen in dreams or visions. You can meditate on the form of a Saint who is free from Raga-Dvesha. 'Yatha Abhimatha Dhyaanaad vaa.' Or, meditate on anything you like best. An aspirant once approached his Guru and asked for instruction on meditation.

The Guru asked him to meditate on Lord Rama. The disciple said: 'I find it very difficult to meditate on Lord Rama.' 'Why?' 'Because I have got inordinate affection for my buffalo.' Then the Guru said: 'Then meditate on the picture of a buffalo.' The disciple sat in deep meditation. One, two, three days passed. The Guru called on the disciple to come out. The disciple said: 'I am not able to come out. I am myself a buffalo. I cannot pass through the door.' The Guru found out that the disciple had perfect concentration of mind. He then gave him the form of Lord Vishnu to meditate upon. Then the disciple entered into deep Samadhi.

There are many obstacles on the path. All these obstacles should be got over. Sleep always disturbs the aspirant. Take light food at night; dash cold water on the face when sleep tries to overpower you; stand up, and do Japa standing for some time; practise Bhastrika—these practices will drive off sleepiness during meditation. Chant OM 10 to 12 times. You will be fit for good concentration. You can keep a bright light in your meditation room. You can combine several of these methods; then success is assured. There is another novel method. Tie your tuft of hair to a nail on the wall with the help of a thread. Now meditate. If you feel drowsy, this nail will pull you up.

The moment you sit for meditation all sorts of evil ideas crop up in the mind. You need not be alarmed. You gave them a long rope till now; they have come to fight with you now, because you wish to annihilate them in toto. This is itself a sign of spiritual growth. If you are steady in your Sadhana, all these evil Samskaras will die by themselves. You will be established in meditation and Samadhi.

What are these knots or Granthis? Avidya, Kama and Karma. Original primordial ignorance is Avidya. On account of this ignorance, there arose desire—Kama. In that Pure Absolute, there is no desire. Through desire came action—Karma. Desire is imperfection. You try to seek your happiness in external things. When there is no imperfection, when there is no desire, you will enjoy the bliss of the

Atman. If you can destroy these cravings and desires through regular meditation, then you can cut these Granthis in the twinkling of an eye.

You should meditate regularly at a particular hour of the day. Then the meditating mood will come by itself at that hour. Besides, you should keep up the meditative Bhava throughout the day, by gradual extension. Then you will be tranquil, peaceful, happy and balanced. You will be able to turn more work more efficiently.

Glory of Meditation

You have to meditate now. You have given a definite promise when you were in the womb that you will meditate and realise yourself. You have forgotten your promise. If you practise meditation regularly, a little sleep is quite sufficient. Meditation for a few minutes will give you good sleep later on; meditation itself will refresh you greatly. Keep up the current of meditation while at work also.

If the mind runs towards an object and craves for sense-enjoyment, tell it 'Wait, O Mind! I will give you the bliss of meditation. Please, therefore, O Desire, leave me now.' You can thus wean your mind away little by little. Once you get real peace and bliss by regular meditation in the early morning, then you will find it impossible to take the mind away from the lotus feet of the Lord, and you will not like to miss a day's meditation. Meditate now. Meditate a little now and see whether there is such ineffable peace in meditation or not. Close your eyes and meditate on Krishna, Rama, or Jesus, on OM, or your father, or whatever you like.

Chant Om. Taste the bliss of the inner Atman. You should be regular in meditation. Meditate in the early morning; have another sitting after bath; another in the evening; and one more before you go to bed.

If you are poor to have a separate meditation room, set apart one corner of the room you have for meditation.

Every day side by side, along with your duties, practise meditation. This is your foremost duty. This should not be neglected on any account. Get up at 4 a.m. Practise a little bit of meditation; a little of Kirtan; study of the Gita or other sacred scriptures; and introspection.

Spiritualise all your daily activities. This is very important. Meditating for half an hour in the morning and then doing all sorts of evil actions during the rest of the day will not help you; the Samskaras created by the morning meditation will be wiped out during the day. You must keep up the spiritual current throughout the day.

If you are regular in your meditation, all doubts and difficulties will vanish by themselves.

2. WITHDRAWAL FROM MULTIPLICITY

Self-restraint is the opposite of self-expression. The latter tends towards Pravritti or life in the variegated Samsara, and the former leads to the Highest Integration through Nivritti or stepping back to Truth. The creative diversifying power is turned in and sublimated into the spiritual splendour. The withdrawal from multiplicity and centering oneself in Unity is effected through Self-restraint which is the austere transformation of the creative objective force into the conscious Power that causes the blossoming of the sense of individual finitude into the expanse of objectless consciousness. Variety is the meaning of manifestation. Every individual force is a copy of the limitless creative force and the natural tendency of this energy is to move towards the creation of multiplicity. This is the reason why the control of the action of creativity is found to be difficult in the case of those who are tied to individual physicality. An individual finds it hard to properly direct the cosmic habit unless he takes recourse to process of Spiritual Realisation. A spiritual Sadhaka goes to the source of this objectified energy and compels the force to diffuse itself in the serene Ground—Noumenon. A person who has let loose the flow of the creative force gets entangled in the process of multiple-creation and ever remains away from the knowledge of the Non-Dual Truth of his Eternal Self. This is the root—the background of the universal ethics that self-control is imperative to a seeker after the Absolute Reality.

Those who have discriminatively grasped the spiritual character of human life refrain from the instinctive practice of self-multiplication and devote themselves to the glorious task of directing the potential energy of conscious contemplation on the Spiritual Ideal through the triple transformation of the active, emotional and intellectual aspects of the general human nature. Such integrated persons possess a mighty power of understanding, analysis and meditation. The Chandogya Upanishad says that when purity and Sattva are increased, there is a generation of immense memory which paves the way to the shattering open of the knot of Self. The most intricate technique of the art of Self-realisation is mastered by the genius of an austere person who has learnt to expand his formative power into the plenitude of limitless life. Such austere spiritual beings glow with the lustrous spiritual strength which handles with ease even the most formidable of the diversifying forces of nature. Fear is unknown to them and their divinised energy is centred in the Self to be utilised in transcending the realm of the ego-sense. They establish themselves in the unbroken vow of leaping over phenomenon into the Heart of Existence. Such is the glory of Self-restraint.

The control of the instincts for possessing the objects is the preparation for world-renunciation in the quest of the Ultimate Essence! An abandonment of earthly nature effected by a distaste for particularities is what marks the character of a true austere Sadhaka. He should not enter the household, for, his path leads to Unity and not to the creative social activity. Alone and unfriended should he carry on the duty of Self-integration through unceasing selflessness and remembrance of the Divine Ideal. Selfless service polishes the self and rubs the ego and renders the person fit for the higher life of Dhyana and Brahma-Chintana. A cutting off from association with relatives is necessary, for, Nivritti-Marga does not allow of any transitory connections.

Fitness for Wisdom

One who is fit for receiving Wisdom of the Self shall receive it 'in due time.' Self-effort and passage of time work simultaneously and one cannot be distinguished from the other, for Providence and Personal exertion cannot be separated as they both work simultaneously, and are interdependent. Rather these are only two names for one and the same force of action.

Sri Sankaracharya had already exhorted that one has to undergo the disciplinary stages of Viveka, Vairagya, Sama, Dama, Uparati, Titiksha, Sraddha, Samadhana and Mumukshutva before getting initiated into the mystery of Existence. One should not be initiated into the Truth of the Absolute unless he is found well developed in all these qualities. Nowadays, generally we find that aspirants do not have a strong desire for liberation. They may have a ray of Viveka and Vairagya of a mild variety. But it is very difficult to find an aspirant who cares for nothing but final Emancipation, who treats the whole world and its contents as mere straw, who meditates incessantly upon how to attain Salvation from embodied existence. It is not easy to understand the meaning of Liberation. How can it be possible for raw men of the world to realise the nullity of earthly existence and of worldly activities? Even advanced aspirants sometimes have got a strong desire for doing something wonderful in this world, something which none has done before. Such people cannot have a real desire for liberation. And such people are unfit for receiving Brahma Vidya. It is only the Uttama-Adhikari, the best qualified—who cares for nothing, who is totally indifferent to the ways of the world, who is ever silent and serene due to the dawn of proper knowledge, who is ever the same among the diverse men of the world, who is undisturbed by the distracted activity of the world, who is calm and peaceful, who has withdrawn himself from the bustle of life, who cares not for either death or life, who is unmindful of what is happening in the world, who is careless towards either this or that—who is really fit to receive the Ultimate wisdom of the Absolute. Even if there is the slightest desire lurking inside other than that for the Realisation of the Absolute, that man will not be able to comprehend the true import of the Vedantic instruction by the Spiritual Teacher (Preceptor). He will have thousand doubts and distractions in the mind which will entirely pull him down from Vedantic Meditation. A person should desire for nothing other than the Realisation of Brahman. There should be no other thought throughout the day than of the way of attaining Self-realisation. Every thought, every speech, every action, nay, every breath of the person should illustrate the method of realising the Absolute. Such a person is fit to receive Vedantic Wisdom.

Guide to Meditation

Meditation is the centering of the force of thought on the highest conception of the ideal to be attained. Hence meditation starts with a belief in the reality of a dual existence, for, without such a faith in duality, meditation lapses into a state of the faculty of thinking and contemplation becomes impossible. Meditation starts with duality and ends in the Glorious Consciousness of the Unity of life.

A belief in the degree of truth and reality in being is necessitated by the fact that the whole universe is a gradual materialisation of the Highest Brahman Itself. A completely transcendent being unconnected with the meditator is impossible to be reached. Truth is immanent tool. The object of meditation is very closely connected with the meditator and exists as his very essence and hence the possibility of the realisation of the Infinite. The world is to be made use of as a step in the ladder of ascent of lhe Glory of Transcendental Spiritual Perfection.

The aspirant is, thus, led to the obvious fact that the existing forces of nature are to be made friends with and utilised as help in spiritual Meditation. One cannot easily deny the differences existing between the hard earth, the liquid water, the hot fire, the blowing wind and the empty space, so long as one is conscious of his relational individuality. The changes of weather, the degrees of intelligence in man, the respective demands of the various sheaths of embodied consciousness, exertion, feeling, will, the passions, the joys, the sorrows and ills of life point to the difference that exists in the process of Truth-Manifestation. The Brahman does not manifest itself equally in all things. It manifests greatly in Divine Beings, in Incarnations and in Sages, less in ordinary human beings, lesser still in an inanimate beings. A complete knowledge of the scheme and the methods of the working of Nature will accelerate the process of the Realisation of the Brahman-consciousness through intensified Meditation.

Tops of mountains, sombre cloudy weather and places near vast expanses of water generate and attract atmospheric electricity and, hence, are best suited for meditation as they add to the energy produced during powerful meditation. Vast expanses of space also help meditation. Cramped places obstruct the consciousness of expanded existence and are not helpful to conscious expansion.

The Uttarakhanda is the region where sages and divinities lived and meditated and is, therefore, the best place suited for meditation. The sacred Ganga and the Himalayas diffuse the most exalted spiritual currents helpful for spiritual meditation. The land above Haridwar (the Gateway to the Land of Hari) extending up to the high Himalayan Peaks is the most blessed land meant for meditation. Sages meditated in this region and have left undying spiritual vibrations.

Facing the North or the East is best suited for meditation. There is a powerful magnetic force in the Northern direction. All blessedness is in the Northern direction

The time from 12 midnight to 4 a.m. is best suited for meditation. There is absolute calmness, coolness, peace and an integrating vibration at that time. Darkness makes existence appear as a one Whole Being, whereas light compels one to perceive the multiplicity of the world. Sunlight, or very bright artificial lights like petromax light (gas light) etc., are not good for meditation, for they distract the mind very much. Dark places are most useful for meditation. Moonlight also is useful for meditation.

During meditation powerful electric current is produced in the body. If, while meditating, the hands and legs are stretched out, the current generated is lost into the air through the tips of fingers and toes. One should lock the fingers or be touching the knees and sit in Padma, Siddha, Sukha or Svastika Asana, so that the current may be circulating in the body itself.

The earth has got the power of absorbing and draining away electric energy. Hence, during meditation, one should sit on tiger skin or deer skin to avoid this mishap and to generate more energy.

No concentration is possible when the spinal cloumn is bent, because, the flow of the current of Prana is thereby obstructed. Hence, one should sit erect for meditation.

One should have either enlightened Intelligence or tenacious faith. If both of these are lacking in a person, he cannot gain concentration on the Reality.

Except in very rare cases, no meditation on the Reality is possible without first deriving help from the direct company of an advanced spiritual personage. The exact technique of attuning the self with the Infinite cannot be known except through the company of an experienced saint or sage. Study of books may stimulate activity but the strength to fight with evil comes only through association with men of wisdom.

The most dreadful enemies of meditation are lust and anger. Those two shall destroy even the very vast energy accumulated through long practice. Hence, one should be extremely circumspect about these two negative forces.

When the eyes and the ears are shut, the whole world is shut out from one's experience. Sound and colour constitute the whole universe. When they are not, nothing is.

Indifference to external happenings is the greatest treasure of the meditator. He should not worry whether the world goes on happily or otherwise.

The meditator should consider his individual personality as a mere insignificant nothing. He should be ever contemplating on the Infinite Fullness.

Desire for nothing but the Infinite alone. This is the greatest of all instructions.

3. CONCENTRATION

Mokshapriya said:

O Beloved Master! Now teach me all about concentration in a nutshell.

Swami Sivananda replied:

Concentration is Dharana or fixing the mind steadily on any internal or external object or God or Brahman the Absolute.

The mind is ever wandering. It ever runs towards sensual objects. It ever thinks of sensual objects. It jumps like a monkey from one object to another in the twinkling of an eye. This is its habit or nature.

Steadying the mind through practice of Vairagya (dispassion) and Abhyasa (concentration) is Dharana.

Dharana does not come in a day, a week or a month. It should be practised with intense faith, fiery zeal for a very long time.

Without Brahmacharya, dispassion or non-attachment or desirelessness, no concentration is possible. Energy should not leak through the sensuous holes.

The practice of Yama (Self-restraint) and Niyama (observance) is also essential for attaining success in concentration.

Be steady in your Asana. Regulate and restrain the breath through the practice of Pranayama. withdraw the senses from the sensual objects (Pratyahara). Now you will be able to practise concentration.

If you are established in concentration, O Mokshapriya, meditation and Samadhi will come by themselves.

Concentration is of two kinds, viz. concrete (gross) and abstract (subtle). For a neophyte or a beginner concrete concentration on a form is very necessary. Later on he can take to concentration on an abstract idea such as beauty, purity, peace, bliss, etc.

Concentrate on a black dot on a wall, candle flame, stars, the picture of the Lord, on the Soham breath in the nose, sun, moon, etc.

Regularity in concentration is of paramount importance. O Mokshapriya! Do not miss a day in your practice. Concentrate at a fixed hour, for a definite time. Adjust your diet. Take Sattvic and light diet. Be careful in the selection of your companions. Give up evil company. Have faith and devotion to your Guru and the Lord. You will attain sure success in concentration, O lover of Truth, O Sadhana Dheera!

4. PRACTICE OF CONCENTRATION

Fix the mind on some object either within the body or without. Keep it there steadily for sometime. This is concentration. You will have to practise this daily.

Purify the mind first through the practice of right conduct and then take to the practice of concentration. Concentration without purity of mind is of no avail. There are some occultists who have concentration; but they have no good character. That is the reason why they do not make any progress in the spiritual line. He who has a steady posture and has purified his nerves and the vital sheath by the constant practice of controlling the breath will be able to concentrate easily. Concentration will be intense if you remove all distractions. A true celibate who has preserved his energy will have wonderful concentration.

Some foolish impatient students take to concentration at once without undergoing, in any manner, any preliminary training in ethics. This is a serious blunder. Ethical perfection is a matter of paramount importance.

A scientist concentrates his mind and invents many new things. Through concentration he opens the layers of the gross mind and penetrates deeply into the higher regions of the mind and gets deeper knowledge. He concentrates all the energies of his mind into one focus and throws them out upon the materials he is analysing and finds out their secrets.

He who has gained abstraction (withdrawing the senses from the objects) will have good concentration. You will have to march on the spiritual path step by step and stage by stage. Lay the foundation of right conduct, postures, regulation of breath and abstraction, to start with. The superstructure of concentration and meditation will be successful then only.

You should be able to visualise the object of concentration very clearly even in its absence. You will have to call up the mental picture at a moment's notice. If you have good concentration you can do this without much difficulty. In the beginning stage of practice, you can concentrate on the tick-tick sound of a watch or on the flame of a candle or any other object that is pleasing to the mind. This is concrete concentration. There is no concentration without something to rest the mind upon. The mind can be fixed on any object in the beginning which is pleasant. It is very, very difficult to fix the mind in the beginning on an object which the mind dislikes.

Sit in lotus-pose (Padmasana) with crossed legs. Fix the gaze on the tip of the nose. This is called the nasal gaze. Do not make any violent effort. Gently look at the tip of the nose. Practise for one minute in the beginning. Gradually increase the time to half an hour or more. This practice steadies the mind. It develops the power of concentration. Even when you walk, you can keep up this practice.

Sit in lotus-pose and practise fixing the mind between the two eyebrows. Do this gently for half a minute. Then gradually increase the time to half an hour or more. There must not be the least violence in the practice. This removes tossing of mind and develops concentration. This is known as frontal gaze. The eyes are directed towards the frontal bone of the forehead. You can select either the nasal gaze or the frontal gaze according to your taste, temperament and capacity.

If you want to increase your power of concentration you will have to reduce your worldly activities. You will have to observe the vow of silence every day for two hours or more.

Practise concentration till the mind is well established on the object of concentration. When the mind runs away from the object bring it back again.

When concentration is deep and intense all other senses cannot operate. He who practises concentration for three hours daily will have tremendous psychic power—he will have a strong will power.

There was a workman who used to manufacture arrows. Once he was very busy with his work. He was so much absorbed in his work that he did not notice even a big party of a Raja passing with his retinue in front of his shop. Such must be the nature of your concentration when you fix your mind on God. You must have the one idea of God and God alone. No doubt it takes some time to complete concentration or one-pointedness of mind. You will have to struggle hard to have single-minded concentration.

Even if the mind runs outside during your practice of meditation do not bother much. Allow it to run. Slowly try to bring it to your object of concentration. By repeated practice the mind will be finally focused in your heart, in the Self, the Indweller of your heart—the final goal of life. In the beginning, the mind may run 80 times. Within six months, it may run 70 times. Within a year, it may run 50 times; within two years, it may run 30 times; within five years, it will be completely fixed in the divine consciousness. Then it will not run out at all even if you try your level best to bring it out like the wandering bull which was in the habit of running to the gardens of different landlords for eating grass but which now eats fresh gram and extract of cotton seeds in its own resting place.

Attention plays a prominent part in concentration. He who has developed his power of attention will have good concentration. A man who is filled with passion and all sorts of fantastic desires can hardly concentrate on any object even for a second. His mind will ever be jumping like a monkey. If you want to increase your power of concentration, you will first have to reduce your worldly desires and worldly activities. You will have to observe Mouna (silence) every day for two hours or even more. You should be able to visualise very clearly the object of concentration even in its absence. You must call up the mental picture at a moment's notice. If you have had a good practice in concentration, you can do this without any difficulty.

He who has gained Pratyahara (withdrawing the senses from the objects) will have good concentration. You will have to march in the spiritual path step by step and stage by stage. Lay the foundation of Yama, Niyama, Asana, Pranayama and Pratyahara to start with. The superstructure of Dharana and Dhyana will be successful only then. In the beginning stage of concentration, you can concentrate on the tick-tick sound of a watch or on the flame of a candle or any other object that is pleasing to the mind. This is called concrete concentration. There can be no concentration without something upon which the mind may rest. The mind can be fixed upon a pleasant object. It is very difficult to fix the mind on any object which the mind dislikes. Fix the mind on some object either within the body or outside. Keep it there steady for sometime. This is called "Dharana". You will have to practise this daily. Laya Yoga has its basis on Dharana.

Vedantins try to fix the mind on the Atman. This is their Dharana. Hatha Yogis and Raja Yogis concentrate their mind on the six Chakras. Bhaktas concentrate on their Ishta Devata. Concentration is a great necessity for all the aspirants.

Those who practise concentration evolve quickly. They can do any kind of work with greater efficiency and in no time. What others can do in six hours can be done easily in half an hour by one who has concentrated his mind. Concentration purifies and calms the surging emotions, strengthens the current of thought and clarifies the ideas. Concentration helps a man in his material progress also. He will turn out very good work in his office or business house. What was cloudy and hazy before becomes clearer and definite; what was very difficult before becomes easy now and what was complex, bewildering and confusing before, comes easily within the mental grasp. You can achieve anything by mental concentration. Nothing is impossible for one who has regularly practised concentration. Clairvoyance, clairaudience, mesmerism, hypnotism, thought-reading, music, mathematics and other sciences depend much upon concentration. Just as the laws of gravitation, cohesion, etc., operate in the physical plane, so also definite laws of association, relativity, contiguity, etc., operate in the mental plane or thought-world. Those who practise concentration should thoroughly understand these laws.

When the mind thinks of an object, it may think of its qualities and its parts also. When it thinks of a cause, it may think of its effect also. If you read the sacred scriptures like the Bhagavad Gita or good books like the Vicar of Wakefield several times, you can get new ideas each time. Through concentration you will get inside. Subtle esoteric meaning will flash out in the field of mental consciousness. You will understand the inner depth of philosophical significance. Train the mind in concentrating on various objects, gross and

subtle, of various sizes. In course of time, a strong habit will
be formed. The moment you sit for concentration the mood
will come at once, quite easily. When desires arise in the
mind do not try to fulfil them. Reject them as soon as they
arise. Thus by gradual practice, the desires can be reduced.
The modifications of the mind will also diminish a lot. You
must get rid of all sorts of mental weaknesses, superstitions,
false and wrong imaginations, false fears and wrong
Samskaras. Then only you will succeed in your
concentration.

5. EXERCISES IN CONCENTRATION

I

Ask your friends to show you some playing cards.
Immediately after the exposure, describe the forms you have
seen. Give the number, name, etc., such as clubs king, spade
ten, diamond queen, heart's jack, and so on.

II

Read two or three pages of a book. Then close the book.
Now attend to what you have read. Abandon all distracting
thoughts. Focus your attention carefully. Allow the mind to
associate, classify, group, combine and compare. You will get
now a fund of knowledge and information on the subject.
Mere skipping over the pages inadvertently is of no use.
There are students who read a book within a few hours. If
you ask them to reproduce some important points of the
book, they will simply blink. If you attend to the subject on
hand very carefully, you will receive clear, strong
impressions. If the impressions are strong, you will have
good memory.

III

Sit in your favourite meditative pose about one foot
from a watch. Concentrate on the tick-tick sound slowly;
whenever the mind runs, again and again try to hear the
sound. Just see how long the mind can be fixed continuously
on the sound.

IV

Sit in on your favourite Asana. Close your eyes. Close the ears with your thumbs or plug the ears with wax or cotton. Try to hear the Anahata sounds (mystic sounds). You will hear various kinds of sounds such as flute, violin, kettledrum, thunderstorm, conch, bells, the humming of a bee, etc. Try to hear the gross sounds first. Hear only one kind of sound. If the mind runs, you can shift it from gross to subtle, or from subtle to gross. Generally you will hear sounds in your right ear. Occasionally you may hear in your left ear also. But try to stick to the sound in one ear. You will get one-pointedness of mind. This is an easy way to capture the mind, because it is enchanted by the sweet sound just as a snake is hypnotised by the note of the snake-charmer.

V

Keep a candle flame in front of you and try to concentrate on the flame. When you are tired of doing this, close your eyes and try to visualise the flame. Do it for half a minute and increase the time to five or ten minutes according to your taste, temperament and capacity. You will see Rishis and Devatas, when you enter into deep concentration.

VI

In a lying posture, concentrate on the moon. Whenever the mind runs, again and again bring it back to the image of the moon. This exercise is very beneficial in the case of some persons having an emotional temperament.

VII

In the above manner, you can concentrate on any star you may single out from the millions of stars shining above your head.

VIII

Sit by the side of a river where you can hear a roaring sound like "OM". Concentrate on that sound as long as you like. This is very thrilling and inspiring.

IX

Lie on your bed in the open air and concentrate upon the blue expansive sky above. Your mind will expand immediately. You will be elevated. The blue sky will remind you of the infinite nature of the Self.

X

Sit in a comfortable posture and concentrate on any one of the numerous abstract virtues such as mercy. Dwell upon this virtue as long as you can.

6. THE KEY STONE IN SADHANA

Having checked all other operations of the mind, bring it to bear upon a single point. This gathering together and bringing to bear upon of a force at a given point on any object, idea or act, forms the process of concentration. The concentrated application of a force makes for maximum results with minimum time and effort.

This law is equally applicable to man in all branches of his life's activities. With the utmost concentrated and careful attention the surgeon executes minute operations. The deepest absorption marks the mental state of the technician, the engineer, the architect or the expert painter, engaged in drawing the minute details of a plan, chart or sketch where accuracy is of paramount importance. A like concentration is displayed by the skilled Swiss workman that fashions the delicate parts of watches and other scientific instruments. Thus in every art and science.

The tremendous power that any force develops when collected and directed through a given point is fully recognised. This is seen in the rush of the water at the sluices of dams, in the impelling power of steam from a railway boiler. As the sunlight when passed through a lens emerges as a single fiery ray of intense power, the whole mind attains a single-pointedness through Dharana. Now experience has shown that interest and attention of the mind is attracted by three distinct means viz. sound, vision (physical or mental) and imagination or idea. The Yogi enters into deep meditation by concentrating his mind upon the mystic inner sound of Pranava. This is the Anahata Nada which becomes audible when the inner sheaths are perfectly purified and harmony established; or again a Mantra is repeated in a harmonious tone and the mind is concentrated on the continuous unbroken sound. A concrete form of any aspect of the deity or the syllable OM is chosen for fixing the mind. The rational and Vedantic type fills the mind with some sublime idea or formula upon which the mind is made to dwell intensely and continuously.

During concentration the mind becomes calm, serene and steady. The various rays of the mind are collected and focussed on the object of meditation. The mind is centred on the Lakshya. There will be no tossing of the mind. One idea occupies the mind. The whole energy of the mind is concentrated on that one idea. The senses become still. They do not function. When there is deep concentration, there is no consciousness of the body and surroundings. He who has good concentration can visualise the picture of the Lord very clearly within the twinkling of the eye.

Manorajya (building castles in the air) is not concentration. It is wild jumping of the mind in the air. Do not mistake Manorajya for concentration or meditation. Check this habit of the mind through introspection and self-analysis.

Meditation in Different Paths

There are different kinds of meditation. A particular kind is best suited to a particular mind. The kind of meditation varies according to taste, temperament, capacity and type of mind of the individual. A devotee meditates on his tutelary deity or Ishta Devata. A Raja Yogi meditates on the special Purusha or Ishvara who is not touched by the afflictions, desires and Karmas. A Hatha Yogi meditates on the Chakras and their presiding deities. A Jnani meditates on his own Self or Atman. You yourself will have to find out the kind of meditation that is suitable for you. If you are not able to do this, you will have to consult a teacher or preceptor who has attained Self-realisation. He will be able to know the nature of the mind and the correct method of meditation for you.

A Raja Yogi enters into the meditative mood deliberately by practising Yama, Niyama, Asana, Pranayama, Pratyahara and Dharana. A Bhakta enters into the meditative mood by cultivating pure love for God. A Vedantin or a Jnana Yogi enters into the meditative mood by acquiring the four means and hearing the Srutis and reflecting on what he has heard. A Hatha Yogi enters into the meditative mood by practising deep and constant Pranayama.

Regular meditation opens the avenues of intuitional knowledge, makes the mind calm and steady, awakens an ecstatic feeling and brings the Yogic student in contact with the source or the Supreme Purusha. If there are doubts, they are all cleared by themselves when you march on the path of Dhyana Yoga steadily. You will yourself feel the way to place your footstep on the next rung of the spiritual ladder. A mysterious inner voice will guide you. Hear this attentively.

When you enter into deep meditation, you will easily rise above consciousness of your body and surroundings. You will have equanimity of mind. You will not be easily distracted. There will be stoppage of upgoing and down-going sensation. The consciousness of egoism will also gradually vanish. You will experience inexplicable joy and indescribable happiness. Gradually reasoning and reflection also will cease.

When you enter the silence through deep meditation, the world outside and all your troubles will drop away. You will enjoy supreme peace. In this silence is supreme light. In this silence is undecaying bliss. In this silence is real strength and joy. The entire system is renewed and invigorated in the depths of Dhyana.

Faith (Shraddha) or confidence is the power of Yoga. Power (Veerya) for the concentration of mind, memory (Smriti) for contemplation, Prajna, discernment, for the direct perception brought about by meditation becomes the means for the attainment of Samadhi, the final limb of Yoga.

The Factor of Grace

But the final leap across the barrier of relativity piercing the evil between the individual and the Absolute is ultimately a question of Divine Grace. Surrender draws down grace. The individual becomes one with the cosmic will through surrender. Grace makes the surrender complete. Without grace perfect union is not possible. Surrender and grace are interrelated. Grace removes all obstacles, snares and pitfalls of the spiritual path.

The Bhakta gets Bhava Samadhi and Mahabhava. He enjoys the warm embrace of the Divine. He attains Divine Aishvarya. All the spiritual wealth of the Lord belongs to him. He is endowed with divine vision or Divya Chakshu. He is endowed with Divya (lustrous) subtle body and Divya (divine) senses. He does not like to have complete absorption or merging in the Lord. He wants to remain himself separate in front of Him and taste the divine honey of Prema. The absorption in the Lord comes to him temporarily in the intensity of his love and experience in the beginning though he does not like it. He attains similarity with God. He is God-like in the beginning. Eventually he attains Sayujya or Oneness.

Samadhi and Deep Sleep

The difference between the non-dual resting and the profound slumber consists in the merging of the mental function in ignorance in the latter and the merging of the same function in the extremely tangible Brahman in the former; the felicity of the latter is enveloped in ignorance, while the blissfulness of Brahman perceived in the former is entirely devoid of covering.

Just as the fire is absorbed into its source when the fuel is burnt out, so also is the mind absorbed into its source, the Atman, when all Sankalpas or thoughts are annihilated. Then only one attains Kaivalya or the state of Absolute Independence. All thoughts cannot be destroyed in a day. The Process of destruction of mental modifications is a difficult and long one. You should not give up the practice of destroying the thoughts half-way, when you come across some difficulties or stumbling blocks. Your first attempt should be the reduction of thoughts.

Reduce your wants and desires first. All thoughts will decrease. Gradually all thoughts will be extirpated. Thoughts are like the waves of the ocean. They are countless. You may become desperate in the beginning. Some thoughts will subside, while some others will gush out like a stream. The same old thoughts that were once suppressed may again show their faces after some time. Never become despondent on any account at any stage of the practice. You will surely get inner spiritual strength. You are bound to·succeed in the end. All the Yogis of yore had to encounter the same difficulties that you are experiencing now.

7. MEDITATION

Meditation is of two kinds viz. concrete meditation and abstract meditation. In concrete meditation the Yogic student meditates on the form of the Lord, Lord Krishna, Lord Rama, Lord Siva, Lord Hari, Gayatri or Devi. In abstract meditation he concentrates the whole energy of the mind on one idea of God or Atman and avoids comparisons of memories and all other ideals. The one idea fills the whole mind. Concentration is fixing the mind on a point or object either internal (in the body) or external (any outside subject). Meditation follows concentration.

Practise meditation in the early morning from 4 to 6. This is the best time for the practice of meditation. Always choose that part of the day or night when your mind is clear and when you are least likely to be disturbed. You can also have a sitting just before retiring to bed. The mind will be calm at this time. You can have good meditation on Sundays, because this is a holiday and the mind is free. Do vigorous meditation on Sundays. You can have good meditation when you live on milk and fruits or fruits alone or when you fast.

Use your commonsense always and try to bring a good turnout in meditation.

You will be able to enter into deep meditation only if you lead a moral life. When you have led the moral life, you may try further to build up discrimination and the other steps in your mind. You can cultivate the mind in concentration and you can finally devote yourself to meditation The more you lead the moral life the more you meditate and the greater likelihood will then be for you to enter into Nirvikalpa Samadhi which can liberate you from the round of births and deaths and can confer on you eternal Bliss and Immortality.

To practise meditation or contemplation in a mind unprepared by non-adherence to the moral precepts is like trying to build a house on rotten foundation. You may build the house, but it will surely fall. You may practise meditation for years, but you will not realise any tangible result or fruit; if you have no ethical foundation, you will fall down. Therefore, mental purity through ethical training is of paramount importance if you wish to achieve success in meditation and Samadhi. Before you attempt to practise meditation, you must have the necessary right understanding. Then only you will have sanguine success in meditation. Much more time is required in the preparation of the mind for meditation than for the actual practice.

The mind is a mischievous imp. It is like a jumping monkey. It must be disciplined daily. Then it will gradually come under your control. It is only by the practical training of your mind that you can prevent bad thoughts and actions from arising and can prevent bad thoughts and actions that have arisen from recurrence. It is only by practical training of your mind that you can encourage good thoughts and actions to arise and can maintain good thoughts and actions when they have arisen.

Just as you require food for the body, so also you require in the shape of prayers, Japa, Kirtan, meditation, etc. food for the Soul. Just as you are agitated when you do not get food in time, so also you will be agitated when you do not pray in the morning and evening at the proper time, if you keep up the practice of prayer and Japa for some time. The soul also wants its food at the proper time. The food for the soul is more essential than the food for the body. Therefore do your prayers, Japa and meditation regularly.

If you do not clean a plate daily, it will lose its lustre. It is the same with the mind, too. The mind becomes impure, if it is not kept clean by the regular practice of meditation. Meditation removes the dross from the mind in an effective manner. Therefore practise meditation in the early morning regularly.

When you sit for meditation, thoughts of your friends and office work, memory of the conversation that took place the previous evening with your friends and relatives will disturb your mind and cause distraction. You will have to withdraw the mind again and again cautiously from these extraneous worldly thoughts and fix it again and again on your Lakshya or point. You will have to disregard and ignore worldly thoughts. Be indifferent. Do not welcome these thoughts. Do not identify yourself with these thoughts or ideas. Say within yourself, "I do not want these thoughts, I have nothing to do with these thoughts". They will vanish gradually.

The external objects are continuously acting upon the brain. The sense-impressions reach the brain through the sense-avenues and produce mental stimuli. Now you are conscious of the external objects. Consciousness may be caused by an awakening either by an external stimulus i.e. a stimulus from a sense-impression or an internal stimulus through memory. Each simple sense-impression is a highly complex bundle of afferent stimuli. "Afferent stimuli" means stimuli that are carried from outside towards the brain. A stimulus is an awakening in the substratum of the mind. The associations of awakenings which arise from a single sense-impression are very complex.

When you meditate, disregard the substratum awakenings in the mind that arise out of the senses. Avoid carefully the comparisons with all other cross references and memories of ideas. Concentrate the whole energy of the mind on the one idea of God or Atman itself without any comparison with any other idea.

Avoid all other sense-impressions and ideas. Prevent the complications that arise out of correlated action in the substratum of the mind. Abstract the mind on the one idea alone. Shut out all other processes of mentation. Now the whole mind will be filled with the one idea only. Nishtha will ensure. Just as the recurrence or repetition of a thought or action leads to perfection of that thought or action, so also does recurrence of the same process, the same idea, leads to the perfection of abstraction, concentration and meditation.

Watch your mind always very carefully. Be ever vigilant. Be on the alert. Do not allow waves of irritability, jealousy, anger, hatred and lust to arise from the mind. These dark waves are enemies of meditation, peace and wisdom. Suppress them immediately by entertaining sublime divine thoughts. Evil thoughts that have arisen may be destroyed by generating good thoughts and maintaining them by repeating any Mantra or name of the Lord, by thinking on any form of the Lord, by practice of Pranayama, by singing the names of the Lord, by doing good actions, by dwelling on the misery that arises from evil thoughts, by abstracting the mind, by analysing the origin of the thoughts, by enquiry of "Who am I?" or by the force of the will resolving to suppress evil thoughts. When you attain the state of purity, no evil thoughts will arise in your mind. Just as it is easy to check the intruder or enemy at the initial stage, so also it is easy to overcome an evil thought as soon as it arises. Nip it in the bud. Do not allow it to strike deep root.

Do not cause pain or suffering to any living being from greed, selfishness, irritability or annoyance. Give up anger or ill-will. Give up the spirit of fighting and heated debates. Do not argue. If you quarrel with somebody or if you have a heated debate with anybody, you cannot meditate for three or four days. Your balance of mind will be upset. Much energy will be wasted in useless channels. The blood will become hot. The nerves will be shattered. You must try your level best to keep a serene mind always. Meditation can proceed from a serene mind only. A serene mind is a valuable spiritual asset for you.

You must practise austerity of speech if you really want to attain quick progress in meditation. You must always speak sweet and loving words. You must speak the truth at any cost. You must not speak any harsh word or any indecent word that is calculated to hurt the feelings of others. You should weigh well your words before they are spoken. You must speak a few words only. This is austerity of speech or Vak-Tapas that will conserve energy and give you peace of mind and inner strength.

There are different kinds of meditation. A particular kind is best suited to a particular mind. The kind of meditation varies according to taste, temperament, capacity and type of mind of the individual. A devotee meditates on his tutelary deity or Ishta Devata. A Raja Yogi meditates on the special Purusha or Ishvara who is not touched by afflictions, desires and Karmas. A Hatha Yogi meditates on the Chakras and their presiding deities. A Jnani meditates on his own Self or Atman. You will have to find out yourself the kind of meditation that is suitable for you. If you are not able to do this, you will have to consult a teacher or preceptor who has attained Self-realisation. He will be able to know the nature of your mind and the correct method of meditation for you.

When you enter into deep meditation, you will have no consciousness of your body or surroundings. You will have equanimity of mind. You will not hear any sounds. There will be stoppage of upgoing and down-coming sensations. The consciousness of egoism also gradually will vanish. You will experience inexplicable joy and indescribable happiness. Gradually reasoning and reflection also cease.

There are many valuable methods about the training of the mind which are essential to mental culture, for instance, the training of memory, the cultivation of reflection, discrimination, Vichara or enquiry of "Who am I?" The practice of meditation itself is a potent clarifier of the memory. The practice of memory-culture powerfully helps meditation in the final attainment.

A Yogi who meditates regularly has a magnetic and charming personality. Those who come in contact with him are much influenced by his sweet voice, powerful speech, lustrous eyes, brilliant complexion, strong healthy body, good behaviour, virtuous qualities and divine nature. Just as a grain of salt dropped in a basin of water dissolves and becomes distributed throughout the whole water, just as sweet fragrance of jasmine pervades the air, so also his spiritual aura becomes infiltrated into the minds of others. People draw joy, peace and strength from him. They are inspired by his speech and give elevation of mind by mere contact with him.

You will have to pass through six stages of meditation and finally you will enter into perfect Nirvikalpa Samadhi, the superconscious state. Form-perception will totally vanish. There is neither meditation nor the meditated, now. The meditator and the meditated have become one. You will attain now the highest knowledge and the eternal supreme peace. This is the goal of life. This is the aim of existence. This is the final beatitude of life. You are an enlightened sage or the illumined Jivanmukta now. You are liberated even while living. Hence you are called a Jivanmukta. You are absolutely free from pain, sorrow, fear, doubt and delusion. You have become identical with Brahman. The bubble has become the ocean. The river has joined the ocean and has become the ocean. All differences and distinctions will totally vanish. You will now experience: "I am the Immortal Self. All indeed is Brahman. There is nothing but Brahman."

There is a place where you will neither hear any sound nor see any colour. That place is Param Dhama or Padam Anamaya (painless seat). This is the realm of peace and bliss. There is no body-consciousness here. Here mind finds rest.

All desires and cravings melt away. The Indriyas remain quiet here. The intellect ceases functioning. There is neither fight nor quarrel here. Will you seek this silent abode through silent meditation ? Solemn stillness reigns supreme here. Rishis of yore attained this place only by melting the mind in this silence. Brahman shines here in His native effulgence.

Forget the body. Forget the surroundings. Forgetting is the highest Sadhana. It helps meditation a great deal. It makes the approach to God easier. By remembering God, you can forget all these things.

Taste the spiritual consciousness by withdrawing the mind from the sensual objects and fixing it at the lotus feet of the Lord, who is ever shining in the chambers of your heart. Merge within by practising deep silent meditation. Plunge deep. Swim freely in the ocean of SAT-CHIT-ANANDA. Float in the Divine river of joy. Tap the source. March direct towards the fountain-head of Divine Consciousness and drink the Nectar. Feel the thrill of Divine embrace and enjoy Divine Ecstasy. I shall leave you here. You have attained the state of immortality and fearlessness.

Practise regular systematic meditation in the same hours daily. You will get the meditative mood easily. The more you meditate the more you will have inner spiritual life, wherein mind and Indriyas do not play; you will be very close to the source Atman. You will enjoy the wave of bliss and peace.

All sensual objects will have no attraction for you now. The world will appear to you as a long dream.

Jnana will dawn on you by constant, deep meditation. You will be fully illumined. The curtain of ignorance will drop now. The sheaths will be torn. The body idea will vanish. You will realise the significance of the Mahavakya, 'Tat Twam Asi.' All differences, distinctions, dualities will disappear. You will see everywhere one infinite, illimitable Atman, full of Bliss, Light and Knowledge. This will be a rare experience, indeed. Do not tremble with fear like Arjuna. Be bold. You will be left alone now. There is nothing to see or hear now. There are no senses. It is all pure consciousness only.

Thou art the Atman. Thou art not this perishable body. Destroy the Moha for this filthy body . Do not utter in future "My body." Say, "this instrument." The sun is setting now. It is drawing within all the rays. Now sit for meditation. Again have a dip in the sacred Atmic Triveni within. Collect all the rays of the mind and plunge within, quite deep, into the innermost recesses of the heart. Rest in the ocean of silence. Enjoy the eternal peace. Your old Jivahood is gone now. All limitations have disappeared. If the desires and old cravings try to hiss, destroy them by the rod of Viveka and the sword of Vairagya.

Keep these two with you always for some time till you get Brahmee-Sthiti (fully established in the Atman).

Om is Sat-Chit-Anand. Om is Infinity, Eternity. Sing OM. Feel OM. Chant OM. Live in OM. Meditate on OM.

8. PRACTICE OF MEDITATION

Concentration is fixing the mind on one point. It is called Dharana in Yoga philosophy. Concentration is collectiveness of thought. It is said to be the placing, setting of mind and mental properties fittingly and well, on a single object. That state, by the strength of which mind and mental properties are placed in one object fittingly and well, without wavering, without scattering, is known as concentration. Meditation follows concentration. There is a continuous flow of one idea only.

The characteristic of concentration is not wandering. Its essence is to destroy wavering. Its manifestation is not shaking. The mind of the happy man is concentrated. Happiness of ease is its proximate cause. Concentration is accompanied by ease, even-mindedness and raptures.

You must be regular in your practice of meditation. You must sit daily both morning and night and at the same hour. The meditative mood or Sattvic Bhava will manifest by itself without any exertion. You must sit in the same place, in the same room. Regularity in meditation is a great desideratum and a *sine qua non*. Rapid progress and great success can be attained if regularity is maintained by the practitioner. Even if you do not realise any tangible result in the practice, you must plod on in the practice with sincerity, earnestness, patience and perseverance. You will be crowned with sanguine success after some time. There is no doubt of this. Do not stop the practice even for a day, under any circumstances, even if you are ailing. Meditation is a first class tonic. The wave of meditation will remove all sorts of diseases. It will infuse spiritual strength, new vigour and vitality. It will renovate and completely overhaul the different systems and constitutions. Meditation will give real rest to the body. Be on the alert to catch the Sattvic wave or the meditative mood. If the meditative mood manifests, stop at once work of any kind, reading, etc. Sit for meditation in right earnest.

Pride, self-sufficiency, arrogance, self-assertive Rajasic nature, irritability, curiosity about the affairs of other people, and hypocrisy are all obstacles in meditation. Subtle forms of these Vrittis lurk in the mind. They operate as oceanic undercurrents. Under pressure of Yoga and meditation, various sorts of dirt in the mind come out, just as dirt of a room that is shut up for six months comes out when you carefully sweep. Aspirants should introspect and watch their minds. They should remove them, one by one, by applying suitable, effective methods. Pride is inveterate. Its branches ramify in all directions in the regions of the Rajasic mind. Again and again it manifests, although the wave subsides temporarily for some time. It asserts when opportunities crop up.

If the aspirant has the nature of being offended easily for trifling things, he cannot make any progress in meditation. He should cultivate amiable, loving nature and adaptability. Then this bad habit will vanish. Some aspirants get easily offended if their bad qualities and defects are pointed out. They become indignant and scorn the man who indicates the defects. They think that the man is concocting them out of jealousy and hatred. This is bad. Other people can very easily find out our defects. A man who has no life of introspection, whose mind is of outgoing tendencies (Bhahirmukha Vritti) cannot recognise his own mistakes. The self-conceit acts as a veil and blurs the mental vision. If an aspirant wants to grow, he must admit his defects when pointed out by others. He must try his level best to eradicate them and must thank the man who points out his defects. Then only he can grow in spirituality and meditation.

It becomes a difficult task to eradicate the self-assertive nature. Every man has built his personality from beginningless time. He has given a long rope to the Rajasic mind to have its own ways. This personality has grown very strong. It becomes difficult to bend this personality and make it pliable and elastic. The man of self-assertive nature wants to dominate over others. He does not want to hear the opinions and the reasons advanced by others, even though they are sound, logical and tenable. He has a pair of jaundiced eyes with *Timira* also. He will say: "Whatever I say is correct, whatever I do is correct; the actions and views of others are incorrect." He will never admit his mistakes. He will try his level best to maintain his own whimsical views by crooked arguments and reasonings. If arguments fail he will take to vituperation and hand to hand fight. If people fail to show respect and honour, he is thrown into a state of fury. He is immensely pleased if anybody begins to flatter him. He will tell any number of lies to justify himself. Self-justifications go hand in hand with self-assertive nature. This is a very dangerous habit. He can never grow in meditation and spirituality so long as he has self-assertive nature with the habit of self-justification. The self-assertive man should change his mental attitude. He must develop the habit of looking at matters from the viewpoint of others. He must have a new vision of righteousness and truthfulness. An aspirant should treat respect and honour as offal and censure and dishonour as ornament.

Man finds it difficult to adjust to the ways and habits of others. His mind is filled with prejudice of caste, creed and colour. He is quite intolerant. He thinks that only his views, opinions and ways of living are right, and the views of others are incorrect. The fault finding nature is ingrained in him. He jumps at once to find the faults of others. He has morbid eyes. He cannot see the good in others. He cannot appreciate the meritorious actions of others. He can brag of his own abilities and actions. That is the reason why he has no peace of mind even for a second. That is the reason why he disagrees with all people and cannot keep up the friendship with others for a long time. Aspirants do not make progress in the path, because they too have these defects to a great degree. They should eradicate them completely by developing tolerance, pure love and other Sattvic qualities.

If there are hindrances or obstacles in the path of Yoga, it is difficult. It is a little unpleasant to carry on the practice of concentration and meditation. It is easy in some aspirants as there are no such oppositions. Obstacles can be removed by sincere prayer, Japa of Om or any other Mantra, divine grace or the grace of Guru. Patanjali Maharshi prescribes Japa of Om with Bhava and meaning. *Tajjapas tadarthabhavanam* for the removal of obstacles. Sri Krishna prescribes the remedy *"Macchittah Sarvadurgaani Matprasaadaat tarishyasi*—Fixing thy thought on Me, thou shalt surmount every difficulty by My grace." Gita: Ch. XVIII-58.

If an aspirant in Kashmir meditates upon his Guru or spiritual guide at Uttarkashi in the Himalayas, a definite connection is established between him and the teacher. The Guru radiates power, peace, joy and bliss to the student in response to his thoughts. He is bathed in the powerful current of magnetism. The stream of spiritual electricity flows steadily from one vessel to another. The student can imbibe or draw from his teacher in proportion to his degree of faith in his master. The more the faith, the greater the imbibing or drawing. Whenever the student sincerely meditates upon his teacher, the teacher also actually feels that a current of prayer (sublime thoughts) proceeds from his student and touches his heart. He who has the inner astral sight can clearly visualise a thin line of bright light between the disciple and the teacher, which is caused by the movement of the vibration of Sattvic thoughts in the ocean of Chitta (mental substance).

If you look upon the world from the higher spiritual plane, you will have a clear vision of the world. In that supreme cosmic consciousness, you will have a knowledge of the whole universe. Arjuna describes thus:

"Into Thy gaping mouths they hurrying rush,
Tremendous toothed and terrible to see;
Some caught within the gaps between Thy teeth
Are seen, their heads to powder crushed and ground.
On every side, all swallowing, fiery tongued,
Thou lickest up mankind, devouring all;
Thy glory filleth space; the universe
Is burning, Vishno, with Thy blazing rays."

Just as small insects or fishes move about here and there in a small lake, just as ants crawl about in the wall of a house, so also, all these little human beings move about hither and thither within the body of the Lord. This vision is thrilling and awe-inspiring. You will see millions of undeveloped souls who run about with countless selfish desires, just as the leucocytes and red corpuscles move about in a drop of fresh blood when seen under the microscope. Amidst this multitude of ignorant, undeveloped human beings, you will find a few fully-developed Jeevanmuktas or *Jnanins* or *Yogis,* scattered in different parts of the world, who stand out as big divine flames or beacon lights or torch bearers to guide the ignorant baby-souls and aspirants, just as the lighthouse stands amidst darkness of the night to guide the captain of a steamer. You will also find some sincere, growing, and half-developed aspirants who emanate a small divine flame, who glitter like the stars on a new moon night.

Wonderful is this vision. Magnanimous is this inner Yogic sight, seeing with the new eye of intuition.

Meditation is the keeping up of one idea of God alone always like the continuous flow of oil *(Taila Dhara Vat)*. Yogins call this *Dhyana*. Jnanins term this *'Nididhyasana'*. Bhakta styles this *'Bhajan'*.

Put a piece of iron rod in the blazing furnace. It becomes red like fire. Remove it. It loses its red colour. If you want to keep it always red, you must always keep it on fire. Even so, if you want to keep the mind charged with the fire of Brahmic wisdom, you must keep it always in contact or touch with the Brahmic fire of Knowledge through constant and intense meditation. You must keep up an unceasing flow of the Brahmic consciousness. Then you will have the *Sahaja Avastha* (natural state).

Meditation acts as a powerful tonic. It is a mental and nervine tonic as well. The holy vibrations penetrate all the cells of the body and cure diseases of the body. Those who meditate save the doctor's bills. The powerful soothing waves that arise during meditation exercise a benign influence on the mind, nerves, organs and cells of the body. The Divine energy freely flows like Taila Dhara (flow of oil from one vessel to another) from the feet of the Lord to the different limbs of the Sadhaka's (Bhakta's) body.

If you can meditate for half an hour, you will be able to engage yourself with peace and spiritual strength in the battle of life for one week through the force of this meditation. Such is the beneficial result of meditation. As you have to move with different minds of a peculiar nature in your daily life, get the strength and peace from meditation and you will have no trouble and worry then.

You will find very often these terms in the Gita: *"Ananya Cheta* —not thinking of another"; *'Matchitta,' 'Nitya Yukta'; 'Manmana'; 'Ekagra Mana'; 'Sarva Bhava'*. These terms denote that you will have to give your full mind, entire 100 per cent mind to God. Then only you will have

Self-realisation. Even if one ray of mind runs outside, it is impossible to attain God-consciousness.

Be silent. Know thyself. Know that. Melt the mind in that. Truth is quite pure and simple.

Asana (posture) steadies the body, Bandhas and Mudras make the body firm. Pranayama makes the body light. Nadi Suddhi produces steadiness of the mind. Having acquired these qualifications you will have to fix the mind on Brahman. Then only meditation will go on steadily with happiness.

The banks of the Ganga or Narmada, the Himalayan scenery, a lovely flower garden, sacred temples—these are the places which elevate the mind in concentration and meditation. Have recourse to them.

A solitary place, spiritual vibratory conditions as at Uttarkasi, Rishikesh, Badri Narayan, a cool place and temperate climate—these conditions are an indispensable requisite for concentration of mind. Just as the salt melts in water, even so the Sattvic mind melts in silence during meditation on Brahman—its Adhishthana (substratum).

When you are a neophyte in meditation, start repeating some Slokas—sublime Slokas or Stotras (hymns) for ten minutes as soon as you sit for meditation. This will elevate the mind. The mind can be easily withdrawn from the worldly objects. Then stop this kind of thinking also and fix the mind on one idea only by repeated and strenuous efforts. Then Nishtha will ensue. You must have a mental image of God or Brahman (concrete or abstract) before you begin to meditate.

When you see the concrete figure of Lord Krishna with open eyes and meditate, it is the concrete form of meditation. When you reflect over the image of Lord Krishna by closing your eyes, it is also concrete form of meditation but it is more abstract. When you meditate on the infinite abstract light, it is still more abstract meditation. The former two types belong to Saguna forms of meditation. The latter to

Nirguna form. Even in Nirguna meditation there is an abstract form in the beginning for fixing the mind. Later on, this form vanishes and the meditator and the meditated become one. Meditation proceeds from the mind.

Examine your character. Pick up some distinct defects in it. Find out its opposite. Let us say that you suffer from irritability. The opposite of irritability is patience. Regularly every morning sit down at 4 in Padma or Siddha Asana in a solitary room for half an hour and begin to think on patience, its value, its practice under provocation, taking one point one day, other on another day, and thinking as steadily as you can, recalling the mind when it wanders. Think of yourself as perfectly patient, a model of patience and end with a vow, "this patience which is my true Self, I will feel and show from today."

For a few days probably there will be no change perceptible. You will still feel and show irritability. Go on practising steadily every morning. Presently as you see an irritable thing, the thought will flash into your mind unbidden: "Should have been patient." Still go on in practice. Soon the thought of patience will arise with the irritable impulse and the outer manifestation will be checked. Still go on practising. The irritable impulse will grow feebler and feebler until you find that irritability has disappeared and the patience has become your normal attitude towards annoyances. In this manner you can develop various virtues as sympathy, self-restraint, purity, humility, benevolence, nobility, generosity, etc.

It is the actions of the mind that are truly termed as Karmas. True liberation results from the disenthralment of the mind. Those who have freed themselves from the fluctuation of their minds come into the possession of the Supreme Nishtha (meditation). Should the mind be purged of all its impurities then it will become very calm and all the Samsaric delusion attended with its births and deaths will soon be destroyed.

Concentration of the mind on God after purification can give you real happiness and knowledge. You are born for this purpose only. You are carried away to external objects through Raga and Moha (attachment and infatuated love). Concentrate upon God in the heart. Dive deep. The Divine Flame, the Light of lights is burning there. Plunge deep. Merge within.

If you place a big mirror in front of a dog and keep some bread in front of the dog, it at once barks by looking at its reflection in the mirror. It foolishly imagines that there is another dog. Even so, man sees his own reflection only through his mind mirror in all the people but foolishly imagines like the dog that they are all different from him and fights on account of hatred and jealousy.

When you start a fire, you heap up some straw, pieces of paper and thin pieces of wood. The fire sometimes gets extinguished quickly. You blow it again several times through the mouth or the blow pipe. After sometime it becomes a small conflagration. You can hardly extinguish it now even vith great effort. Even so in the beginning of meditation neophytes fall down from meditation into their old grooves. They will have to lift up their minds again and again and fix on the Lakshya. When the meditation becomes deep and steady, they get established in God eventually. Then the meditation becomes *Sahaja* (natural). It becomes habitual.

9. FRUITS OF MEDITATION

Neophytes should remember again and again some important Vedantic Texts daily. Then only his doubts will be removed. Then only he will be established in the path. These texts are: "Being only was in the beginning, One without a second" Chhandogya Upanishad VI-2-1. "In the beginning all this was one Self only" Aitareya Upanishad VI-2-l. "This is the Brahman, without cause and without effect; this Self is Brahman perceiving everything" Brihadaranyaka Upanishad II-5-19, "That immortal Brahman before" Mandukya Upanishad, II-2-7.

Concern yourself with the present only. Do not look back upon the past or the future. Then alone you will be really happy. You will be free from cares, worries and anxieties. You will have a long life. Destroy the *Sankalpas* through strenuous efforts. Meditate ceaselessly upon that *Satchidananda* Brahman and attain the Supreme immaculate state. May you prosper gloriously ! May you live drowned in the ocean of Brahmic bliss in an illumined state !

This immortal Atman cannot be attained without constant practice. Therefore, he who wishes to attain immortality and freedom should meditate on the Self or Brahman for a long time.

The real solitary place is Brahman who is one without a second. There is neither sound nor colour here. There is no disturbance of any sort here. The only companion for you in the beginning of your practice is Brahman. When you become That during deep meditation, you are left alone (Sivah Kevaloham).

Atman is the fountain-source of energy. Thinking on Atman or the source for energy also is a dynamic method for augmenting energy, strength and power.

If you once think for even a second of the all-pervading pure, immortal, Satchidananda Atman or Brahman, this is tantamount to taking thousand and eight dips in the sacred Triveni—the Junction of holy rivers at Prayag. This is the real mental sacred bath. Physical bath is nothing when compared to this internal bath of wisdom or knowledge.

Worship God or Atman with the flowers of Jnana, contentment, peace, joy and equal vision. This will constitute real worship. Offerings of rose, jasmine, sandal paste, incense, sweetmeats and fruits are nothing when compared to the offerings of Jnana, contentment, etc. These are the offerings given by ignorant persons.

Try to identify yourself with the eternal, immortal, ever pure Atman or soul that resides in the chambers of your heart. Think and feel always: "I am the very pure Atman."

This one thought will remove all troubles and fanciful thoughts. The mind wants to delude you. Start this anticurrent of thought. The mind will lurk like a thief. Be careful.

10. MEDITATION ON OM

Retire into the meditation chamber. Sit on Padma, Siddha, Svastika or Sukha Asana to begin with. Relax the muscles. Close the eyes. Concentrate the gaze on Trikute, the space between the two eyebrows. Repeat OM mentally with Brahman Bhavana. This Bhavana is a *sine qua non*, very very important. Silence the conscious mind.

Repeat mentally, feel constantly,

All-pervading Ocean of Light I am	Om Om Om!
Infinity I am	Om Om Om!
All-pervading infinite Light I am	Om Om Om!
Vyapaka Paripoorna Jyotirmaya	Om Om Om!
Brahman I am	Om Om Om!
Omnipotent I am	Om Om Om!
Omniscient I am	Om Om Om!
All bliss I am	Om Om Om!
Satchidananda I am	Om Om Om!
All purity I am	Om Om Om!
All glory I am	Om Om Om!

All Upadhis will be sublated. All Granthis (heart-knots, ignorance) will be cut asunder. The thin veil, Avarana, will be pierced. The Pancha Kosha Adhyasa (superimposition) will be removed. You will rest doubtless in Satchidananda state. You will get the highest knowledge, highest bliss, highest realisation, and highest end of life. *"Brahma vit Brahmaiva Bhavati."* You will become Suddha Satchidananda Vyapaka Paripoorna Brahman. *"Nasti Atra Samsaya"* there is no doubt of that, here.

There is no difficulty at all in the Atma Darshan. You can have this within the twinkling of an eye as Raja Janaka had, before you can squeeze a flower with fingers, within the time taken for a grain to fall when rolled over a pot. You must do earnest, constant and intense practice. You are bound to succeed in two or three years.

Nowadays there are plenty of "Talking Brahmans." No flowery talk or verbosity can make a man Brahman. It is constant, intense, earnest *Sadhana* alone that can give a man direct Aparoksha Brahma realisation *(Svanubhava* or *Sakshatkara)* wherein he sees the solid Brahman just as he sees the solid white wall in front of him, just as he feels the table behind him.

11. INSTRUCTIONS ON MEDITATION

Mokshapriya said:

O Blessed Teacher, now instruct me on Meditation. My mind is ever wandering despite my effort in the early morning during Brahmamuhurta—4 a.m.

Swami Sivananda replied:

O Mokshapriya, hearken to me with rapt attention and one-pointed mind. *Dhyanam nirvishayam manah:* meditation is freeing the mind from thoughts of sense-objects. Mind dwells on God and God alone during meditation.

All on a sudden you cannot jump to meditation and Samadhi. You will fall down and break your legs. Can a student of Third Form understand the "Theory of Relativity", "Advanced Mathematics", etc.?

Purify your heart first through selfless service, recitation of Lord's names, Pranayama, etc. Get yourself established in Sadachara or right conduct. Have perfect ethical perfection. Then alone will you be established in deep meditation.

Meditation follows concentration and Samadhi follows meditation.

A gross mind, O friend, O Mokshapriya, wants a concrete object for meditation, in the beginning. Meditation on a concrete form such as the form of Lord Krishna with flute in hand, or the form of Lord Jesus or Lord Buddha is very necessary in the beginning. This is Saguna meditation or meditation on the form of the Lord with attributes.

Think of His attributes such as Omnipresence, Omniscience, Omnipotence, purity and perfection, etc. when you meditate on His form.

Gradually the mind will be prepared and disciplined to take up the higher Nirakara and Nirguna meditation, formless and attributeless meditation on the Pure Nirguna Brahman.

Deep meditation cannot come in a day or a week or a month. You will have to struggle hard for a long time. Be patient. Be persevering. Be vigilant and diligent. Get rid of all Vasanas, cravings and ambitions. Cultivate burning dispassion, burning aspiration or longing for Self-realisation. Gradually you will enter into deep meditation.

Struggle, O Mokshapriya, struggle again. Strive hard. Meditate. Meditate. Meditate. You will surely attain success in the end. Mark my word, O spiritual hero!

12. OBSTACLES IN MEDITATION

Mokshapriya said:

O Lord! Please tell me now what are the obstacles in meditation.

Swami Sivananda replied:

O Mokshapriya! Just listen with rapt attention. The chief obstacles are Laya (sleep), Vikshepa (tossing of mind), Kashaya (Vasanas or subtle, hidden desires), Rasasvada (bliss of Savikalpa Samadhi), lack of Brahmacharya, spiritual pride, laziness, disease, company of worldlings, overeating, overwork, too much mixing with people, and self-assertive Rajasic nature.

Conquer sleep through Pranayama, Asanas and light diet.

Remove Vikshepa through Pranayama, Japa, Upasana or worship, Trataka, etc.

Destroy Kashaya through dispassion, discrimination, study of books which treat of dispassion, meditation, enquiry, etc.

Rasasvada is the bliss which one gets during the experience of lower Savikalpa Samadhi. This is also an obstacle in meditation, because the Yogi gets false contentment, imagines that he has reached the highest Nirvikalpa state, stops his Sadhana and does not attempt to attain the highest state. Rise above Rasasvada; struggle and reach the Nirvikalpa Samadhi.

Failure in Brahmacharya fills the mind with impurity, increases the lease of mundane life here and strengthens the sexual Vasana. Therefore, observe unbroken celibacy.

When the aspirant gets some spiritual progress, he develops spiritual pride. He thinks that he is superior to the householders. Maya assumes various forms. Destroy the spiritual pride through self-analysis and enquiry.

Laziness is another obstacle. Practise Asanas and Pranayamas. Do vigorous selfless service for two hours daily. Run. Draw water from the well. Carry stones. Laziness will disappear.

Observe the laws of health and hygiene. Practise regular exercises, Asanas, Pranayamas. Be moderate in eating and drinking, etc. You will enjoy good health.

Shun the company of worldly persons who always talk on sexual matters, money and worldly things.

Do not overwork. This will produce fatigue. You cannot meditate.

Do not mix much with people. Raga-Dvesha (likes and dislikes) will increase. The mind will be perturbed.

Kill the self-assertive Rajasic nature through humility, enquiry, reflection and meditation. Be vigilant. Fill the mind with Sattva.

O Mokshapriya! Remove the obstacles one by one. March on boldly in the spiritual path and reach the goal quickly.

13. EXPERIENCES IN MEDITATION

Mokshapriya said:

Guru Maharaj! What will be the experiences in meditation?

Swami Sivananda answered:

Experiences differ in Sadhakas according to the nature of their Sadhana and the Yoga they are practising. The highest experience, Nirvikalpa Samadhi, is the same in all aspirants.

Hatha Yogis and Laya Yogis hear Anahata Sounds. They are gross and subtle. Sometimes they hear the sounds of bells, the sounds of drums, the sound of flute, lute, Vina. Sometimes they hear thunder, the sound of Mridanga, etc.

Some Raja Yogis see brilliant lights during meditation in the Ajna, the space between the two eyebrows. They are like the sun, moon, stars, pin-points. Sometimes they see coloured lights, green, blue, red, etc.

Sometimes they see rivers, mountains, landscapes, blue sky. They get the vision of Rishis, Munis, etc. They behold their own faces.

Advanced Yogis experience Cosmic Consciousness. This is a rare experience.

Some float in the air. The subtle, astral body gets detached from the physical body. They have astral journey, and move about in the astral world.

Bhaktas get Darshan of their Ishta or tutelary deity.

Advanced Bhaktas go to Brahma Loka, Vaikuntha and Kailas.

A Jnana Yogi passes through the stages of darkness, light sleep and Moha and reach eventually the stage of Nirvikalpa Samadhi.

The bliss of Nirvikalpa Samadhi cannot be expressed in words O Mokshapriya! You will have to experience it yourself in Samadhi. The bliss of Savikalpa Samadhi is much inferior to that of Nirvikalpa Samadhi.

14. SLEEP AND SAMADHI

Mokshapriya said:

O Purushottama, I have now understood the nature and essence of Samadhi. May I know the difference between sleep and Samadhi.

Swami Sivananda answered:

Well said, O Mokshapriya; this is indeed a beautiful question. I shall give you the reply:

Sleep is a Jada or inert state. But Samadhi is a state of pure awareness or pure consciousness.

When a man returns from sleep he has no experience of the transcendental wisdom of the Self. He is heavy and dull. But when the Yogi or Sage comes down from his state of Samadhi he is full of supreme transcendental wisdom of Atman. He can clear all your doubts. He will inspire and elevate you. He is Brahman Himself.

Samadhi is sleepless sleep. The sage has no consciousness of external world. He is drowned in the ocean of bliss and wisdom.

O Mokshapriya, in sleep there is deep Tamas. The individual soul rests in Karana Sareera or causal body. In Samadhi he rests in Brahman or Satchidananda Svaroopa.

If you wake up, deep sleep state disappears. Therefore a changing state is illusory or unreal. But the Samadhi or the superconscious state is the witnessing Consciousness of the three states. It always exists. Therefore it is the only real State.

In sleep the Vasanas and Samskaras are in a very subtle state. But in Samadhi they are burnt in toto by the fire of wisdom.

Burn the egoism and Vasanas, and the five senses, and enjoy the eternal Bliss of this sleepless Sleep, O Mokshapriya.

15. SAMADHI

Mokshapriya said:

Blessed Swamin! I have a clear understanding now of the previous Angas or limbs of Yoga. What is Samadhi, then?

Swami Sivananda answered:

O Mokshapriya! This is the most difficult matter for explanation. Words and language are imperfect to describe this exalted state.

Samadhi is superconscious state or union with Brahman or the Absolute. Mind, intellect and the senses cease functioning. They are absorbed in Mula Prakriti or the Primordial matter.

It is a state of eternal Bliss and eternal Wisdom. All dualities vanish in toto here.

You will have to experience this state yourself through direct intuitive cognition. Can you explain the taste of sugar-candy or the conjugal happiness to anybody?

Samadhi is subjective consciousness of Brahman. All visible objects merge in the invisible or the Unseen. The individual soul becomes that which he contemplates.

The experience of a Raja Yogi and a Bhakta is dualistic in the beginning. Later on they too experience the non-dual Bliss of Supreme Brahman.

There are two kinds of Samadhi, viz. Savikalpa and Nirvikalpa. In Savikalpa Samadhi there is one idea, there is the Triputi or the triad, knower, knowledge and knowable. In Nirvikalpa Samadhi the triad vanishes. There is not a single idea.

O Mokshapriya, some ignorant aspirants mistake deep sleep and Tamas for the state of Samadhi. They pose for Samadhists by closing their eyes. Samadhi is perfect Self-awareness. It is extremely difficult to enter the state of Samadhi.

Tossing of mind, sleep, cravings, carelessness, indecision, subtle Vasanas, the happiness of Savikalpa Samadhi, doubt, spiritual pride, institutional egoism, etc. are all obstacles to the attainment of Nirvikalpa Samadhi.

O Mokshapriya! Struggle hard. Obtain the Grace of Guru and Ishvara. Live in seclusion. Meditate ceaselessly. You will enjoy the Supreme Bliss of Samadhi.

16. DHYANA YOGA ACCORDING TO YOGASARA UPANISHAD

MANTRA

Dharana or concentration is fixing the mind on an idea or a point or object either internal or external.

Notes and Commentary

It is very difficult to say where concentration ends and meditation begins. Meditation follows concentration.

Concentration is steadfastness of mind. If you remove all causes of distraction, your power of concentration will increase. A true Brahmachari who has preserved his Veerya will have wonderful concentration. Attention plays a prominent part in concentration. He who has developed his power of attention will have good concentration. You should be able to visualise very clearly the object of concentration even in its absence. You must call up the mental picture in a moment's notice. If you have good practice in concentration you can do this without difficulty. He who has gained success in Pratyahara (abstraction) by withdrawing the Indriyas from the various objects will have good concentration. You will have to march in the spiritual path step by step, stage by stage. Lay the foundation of Yama (right conduct), Niyama, Asana (posture), Pranayama and Pratyahara to start with. The superstructure of Dharana (concentration), Dhyana (meditation) and Samadhi will be successful then only.

Asana is Bahiranga Sadhana (external); Dhyana is Antaranga Sadhana (internal). When compared with Dhyana and Samadhi, even Dharana is Bahiranga Sadhana. He who has steady Asana and has purified the Yoga-Nadis and the Pranamaya Kosha (vital sheath) through Pranayama will be able to concentrate easily. You can concentrate internally on any of the seven plexus or Chakras or centres of spiritual energy viz., Muladhara, Svadhisthana, Manipura, Anahata, Visuddha, Ajna and Sahasrara, or at the tip of the nose or tip of the tongue or externally on the picture of any Devata, Hari, Hara, Krishna or Devi. You can concentrate on the tick-tick sound of a watch or on the flame of a candle or on a black point on a wall or a pencil or rose flower or any pleasing object. This is concrete concentration (Sthoola). There can be no concentration without something upon which the mind may rest. The mind can be fixed easily on a pleasing object such as jasmine flower, mango or orange or a loving friend. It is difficult to fix the mind in the beginning on any object which it dislikes such as faecal matter, cobra, enemy, ugly face, etc. Practise concentration till the mind is well established on the object of concentration. When the mind runs away from the object of concentration bring it back again and again to the object. Lord Krishna says in the Gita: *"Yato Yato nischarati manas chanchalam asthiram, Tatas tato niyamya etat atmanyeva vasam nayet*—As often as the wavering and unsteady mind goes forth, so often, reining it in, let him bring it under the control of the Self."

If you want to increase your power of concentration you will have to reduce your worldly activities (Vyavahara Kshaya). You will have to observe Mouna also (vow of silence) for two hours daily. A man whose mind is filled with passion and all sorts of fantastic desires can hardly concentrate on any object even for a second. His mind will be jumping like a balloon. Regulate and master the breath. Subdue the senses and then fix the mind on any pleasing object. Associate the ideas of holiness and purity with the object.

You can concentrate on the space between the two eyebrows (Trikuti). You can concentrate on the mystic sounds (Anahata Dhvani) that you hear from your right ear.

You can concentrate on OM picture. The picture of Lord Krishna with flute in hand and the picture of Lord Vishnu with conch, discus, mace and lotus are very good for concentration. You can concentrate on the picture of your Guru or any saint also. Vedantins try to fix the mind on Atman, the inner Self. This is their Dharana.

Dharana is the sixth stage or limb of Ashtanga Yoga or Raja Yoga of Patanjali Maharshi. In Dharana you will have only one Vritti or wave in the mind-lake. The mind assumes the form of only one object. All other operations of the mind are suspended or stopped. He who can practise real concentration for half or one hour will have tremendous psychic powers. His will also will be very powerful.

When Hatha Yogis concentrate their minds on Shadadhar or the six supports (the Shad-chakras), they concentrate their minds on the respective presiding Devatas also viz. Ganesh, Brahma, Vishnu, Rudra, Ishvara and Sadasiva. Control the breath through Pranayama. Subdue the Indriyas through Pratyahara. And then fix the mind either on Saguna or Nirguna Brahman. According to Hatha-Yogic school, a Yogi who can suspend his breath by Kumbhaka for 20 minutes can have very good Dharana. He will have a very tranquil mind. Pranayama steadies the mind, removes Vikshepa (distraction) and increases the power of concentration. Those who practise Kechari Mudra by cutting the *frenum linguae* and lengthening the tongue and fixing it in the hole in the palate by taking upwards will have good Dharana.

Those who practise concentration evolve quickly. They can do any work with scientific accuracy and great efficiency. What others do in six hours can be done by one who has concentration within half an hour. What others can read in six hours, can be read by one who has concentration within half an hour. Concentration purifies and calms the surging emotions, strengthens the current of thought and clarifies the ideas. Concentration helps a man in his material progress also. He will have a very good turnout of work in his office or business house. What was cloudy and hazy before becomes clear and definite. What was difficult before becomes easy now and what was complex, bewildering and confusing before comes easily within the mental grasp. You can achieve anything through concentration. Nothing is impossible to a man who practises regular concentration. It is very difficult to practise concentration when one is hungry and when one is suffering from an acute disease. He who practises concentration will possess very good health and very clear mental vision.

Retire into a quiet room; sit on Padmasana. Close your eyes. See what happens when you concentrate on an apple. You may think of its colour, shape, size and its different parts such as skin pulp, seeds, etc. You may think of the places (Australia or Kashmir) wherefrom it is imported. You may think of its acidic or sweet taste and its effects on the digestive system and blood. Through law of association, ideas of some other fruits also may try to enter. The mind may entertain some other extraneous ideas. It may begin to wander about. It may think of meeting a friend at the railway station at 4 p.m. It may think of purchasing a towel or a tin of tea and biscuit. It may ponder over some unpleasant happening that occurred the previous day. You must try to have a definite line of thought. There must not be any break in the line of thinking. You must not allow other thoughts which are not connected with the object on hand to enter. You will have to struggle hard to get success in this direction. The mind will try its level best to run in the old grooves and to take its old familiar road or old beaten path. The attempt is somewhat like going uphill. You will rejoice when you get even some success in concentration. Just as laws of gravitation, cohesion, etc. operate in the physical plane, so also definite laws of thought such as law of association, law of relativity, law of continuity, etc., operate in the mental plane or thought-world. Those who practise concentration should thoroughly understand these laws. When the mind thinks of an object, it may think of its qualities and its parts also. When it thinks of a cause, it may think of its effects also.

If you read with concentration the Bhagavad Gita, the Ramayana, or the eleventh Skandha of the Bhagavata several times, you will get new ideas each time. Through concentration you will get penetrative insight. Subtle, esoteric meanings will flash out in the field of mental consciousness. You will understand inner depths of philosophical significance. When you concentrate on any object do not wrestle with the mind. Avoid tension anywhere in the body or mind. Think gently of the object in a continuous manner. Do not allow the mind to wander away.

If emotions disturb you during concentration, do not mind them. They will pass away soon. If you try to drive them, you will have to tax your will-force. Have an indifferent attitude. The Vedantin uses the formulae: "I do not care. Get out. I am a Sakshi (witness of mental modifications)" to drive the emotions. The Bhakta simply prays and help comes from God.

Train the mind in concentration on various subjects, gross and subtle and of various sizes, small, medium and big. In course of time a strong habit of concentration will be formed. The moment you sit in concentration the mood will come at once quite easily. When you read a book, you must read it with concentration. There is no use of skipping over the pages in a hurried manner. Read one page in the Gita. Close the book. Concentrate on what you have read. Find out parallel lines in the Mahabharata, the Upanishads and the Bhagavata. Compare and contrast.

For a neophyte, the practice of concentration is disgusting and tiring in the beginning. He has to cut new grooves in the mind and brain. After some months, he will get great interest in concentration. He will enjoy a new kind of happiness, the concentration-Ananda. He will become restless if he fails to enjoy this new kind of happiness even for one day. Concentration is the only way to get rid of the worldly miseries and tribulations. Your only duty is to practise concentration. You have taken this physical body to practise concentration and through concentration to realise the Self. Charity, Rajasuya-Yajna are nothing when compared to concentration. They are playthings only.

Through Vairagya, Pratyahara and practice of concentration, the dissipated rays of wandering mind are slowly collected. Through steady practice it is rendered one-pointed. How happy and strong is that Yogi who has one-pointed mind! He can turn out voluminous work in the twinkling of an eye.

Those who practise concentration off and on will have a steady mind only occasionally. Sometimes the mind will begin to wander and will be quite unfit for application. You must have a mind that will obey you at all times sincerely and carry out all your commands in the best possible manner at any time. Steady and systematic practice of Raja Yoga will make the mind very obedient and faithful.

There are five Yoga Bhumikas or five stages of the mind viz., Kshipa, Mudha (forgetfulness), Vikshipta (gathering mind), Ekagra (one-pointed), Niruddha (controlled or well restrained). By gradual and well regulated practice of concentration daily, the rays of the wandering mind are collected. It becomes one-pointed. Eventually it is curbed properly. It comes under proper control.

If the aspirant pursues, what is not fitting, his progress is painful and sluggish. He who pursues what is fitting gets easy progress and quick intuition. He who has no past conditions or spiritual Samskaras of previous births makes painful progress. One who has such Samskaras makes easy progress. In one whose nature is actually corrupt and whose controlling faculties are weak, progress is painful and intuition is sluggish. But to one of keen controlling faculties progress is rapid and intuition is quick. In one overcome by ignorance, intuition is sluggish; to one not so overcome, intuition is rapid.

Dhyana or Meditation is the keeping up of flow of one idea like the flow of oil.

Meditation is of two kinds viz., concrete and abstract. If you meditate on any picture of concrete object it is concrete meditation. If you meditate on an abstract idea, on any quality (such as mercy, tolerance) it is abstract meditation. A beginner should practise concrete meditation. For some, abstract meditation is more easy than concrete.

The aspirant can take up the practice of meditation after he is well up in Pratyahara (abstraction of Indriyas) and concentration. If the Indriyas are turbulent, if the mind cannot be fixed on the point, no meditation is possible even within hundreds of years. One should go stage by stage, step by step. The mind should be withdrawn again and again to the point when it runs. One should reduce his wants and renounce all sorts of wild, vain desires of the mind. A desireless man only can sit quiet and practise meditation. Sattvic light diet and Brahmachraya arc the prerequisites for the practice of meditation.

Consciousness is of two kinds viz., focussing consciousness and marginal consciousness. When you concentrate on Trikuti, the space midway between the two eyebrows, your focussing consciousness is on the Trikuti. When some flies sit on your left hand during meditation, you drive them with your right hand. When you become conscious of the flies it is called marginal consciousness.

A seed which has remained in fire for a second will not sprout into leaves even though sown in a fertile soil. Even so a mind that does meditation for some time but runs towards sensual objects on account of unsteadiness will not bring in the full fruits of Yoga.

Samadhi is of two kinds, Samprajnata and Asamprajnata.

Samadhi means superconscious state, wherein the Yogi gets supersensual experiences. Samadhi is of two kinds viz., Samprajnata or Sabija or Savikalpa and Asamprajnata or

Nirbija or Nirvikalpa. In Savikalpa Samadhi there are Triputi or triad—the knower, knowledge and knowable. There is Alambana or support for the mind to lean upon. The Samskaras are not fried. In Nirvikalpa, there is neither Triputi nor Alambana. The Samskaras are fried in toto. The Nirvikalpa Samadhi only can destroy birth and death, and bring the highest knowledge and bliss. Savikalpa Samadhi is of various kinds—Savitarka and Nirvitarka, Savichara and Nirvichara, Saananda and Asmita.

When you get full success or perfection (Siddhi) in Raja Yoga by entering into Asamprajnata Samadhi (Nirvikalpa state) all the Samskaras and Vasanas which bring on rebirths are totally fried up. All Vrittis or mental modifications that arise from the mind-lake come under restraint. The five afflictions viz., Avidya (ignorance) Asmita (egoism), Raga-Dvesha (love and hatred), and Abhinivesa (clinging to life) are destroyed and the bonds of Karma are annihilated. Control the mind and the senses, become desireless, develop the power of endurance, contemplate, see the Self in the Self. Samadhi brings on the highest good (Nisreyas) and exaltation (Abhyudaya). It gives Moksha (deliverance from the wheel of births and deaths). The afflictions, egoism, etc., have their root in Avidya (ignorance). With the advent of the knowledge of the Self, the ignorance vanishes. With the disappearance of the root cause viz., ignorance, egoism, etc., also disappear.

In the Asamprajnata Samadhi, all the modifications of the mind are completely restrained. All the residual Samaskaras also are totally fried up. This is the highest Samadhi of Raja-Yoga. This is also known as Nirbija Samadhi (without seeds) and Nirvikalpa Samadhi.

Dharma Megha in Raja-Yoga means "the cloud of virtue". Just as clouds shower rain, so also this Dharma Megha Samadhi showers on the Yogis omniscience and all sorts of Siddhis or powers. Karma is the seed for life state, life period and life experience. Nirbija Samadhi will burn up all the seeds.

The Vision of a Sage

The Jnani who has full Self-realisation sees all beings in the Self and the Self in all beings. There is nothing other than Brahman for him. He moves about fearlessly in the world.

This is the experience of a realised soul who is resting in his own Svaroopa. This is the vision of an Atma-Jnani. All water-tight compartments have disappeared. He has neither prejudice nor dislike for anything or any person. He is one who has transcended the order and stage of life (Ativarnasrami). He will take food from anybody's hands and sleep wherever he likes. He is not bound by the man-made rules of the society. He is above public opinion. That does not mean he will deviate himself from the rules of conduct. Whatever he does will be in strict accordance with the injunctions of the Sastras. If you ask a man who talked in the dream. "Mr. Surajmal, did you talk anything last night in your dream?" He will say, "No, I did not know anything. I did not talk anything." Similar will be the experience of a Jnani who does actions in the world. It will be like a plaything of a boy. He has dual consciousness of Brahman (like Choranari who does work in her house but whose mind is on her sweet paramour or like the crow which moves the one eye through the two eye-sockets and has vision of this side and that side). He sees the whole world within himself. There is nothing outside for him. On account of the remnant of ignorance (Lesh Avidya), he moves about, eats, drinks, sleeps, etc. Just as the pot in which asafoetida or onion is kept emits the smell a bit even when it is cleaned several times, so also a small trace of ignorance still remains in the mind (Antahkarana) of a Jnani even. That is the reason why he eats and drinks. This is called Lesha Avidya.

17. THE OBSTACLES, ACCORDING TO VEDANTASARA UPANISHAD

Laya, Vikshepa, Kashaya, Rasasvada are the four important obstacles that stand in the way of attaining Self-realisation.

Laya is sleep. The mind that is withdrawn from the sensual objects enters into deep sleep through the force of old Samskaras of deep sleep. The aspirant should try to fix the mind on the Self by not allowing the mind to pass into the state of deep sleep. He must be ever vigilant. If the sleepy condition still persists despite your vigorous efforts, you must find out the causes that induce sleep and then you must remove those causes. Then you should again practise meditation. Indigestion, heavy food, too much walking, insufficient sleep at night are the causes that produce sleep during meditation. If you have disturbed sleep at night you can take a little rest in the afternoon the following day. But do not develop a habit of sleeping in the day. Do not take any food till you get a very keen appetite. Indigestion can be removed by this method. Do not overload the stomach. Practise Mitahara. Get up when three quarters of your stomach is full, when there is slight inclination to take some more food. Train the stomach. Give up too much walking also. Practice of Pranayama also will remove Laya.

The mind that is withdrawn from sleep does not enter into meditation. It again and again thinks of the sensual enjoyments through the force of Samskaras of waking state and struggles hard to attain the desired objects. This is Vikshepa or tossing of mind. You should withdraw the mind again and again from the objects through discrimination and enquiry (Vichara). You should practise Bheda-Drishti, Mithya-Drishti and Dosha-Drishti. You should feel again and again: "This world is unreal (Mithya Drishti). This world never exists (Bheda-Drishti). Sensual enjoyment is the root cause for human sufferings (Dosha-drishti)." You must eradicate Vikshepa by the above method and then practise meditation again and again. Just as a bird that is chased by a hawk goes inside a house and comes out immediately for want of a suitable resting place, so also the mind comes outside to wander about in the sensual objects as it finds it difficult to rest in the very, very subtle Atman. This outgoing tendency of the mind or outgoing Vritti is called Vikshepa.

When the mind is turned inside after eradicating Laya and Vikshepa it refuses to enter into deep meditation. Through the force of strong hidden Vasanas, and strong Raga, it gets attached to objects. It is drowned in sorrow. There is one-pointedness of mind now. This state must not be mistaken for Samadhi. This is Kashaya. This is Manorajya or building castles in the air. The mind thinks of the wife, son and wealth. This is Bahya-Raga (external attachment). It thinks of the past and plans for the future. This is internal attachment (Antar-Raga). You can remove Kashaya by adopting the same methods which you have used for eradicating Vikshepa.

Bahya-Vishayakara Vritti is Vikshepa. That Vritti arises from the force of Samskaras of Raga from within is Kashaya. Kashaya simulates Samadhi. You must be very careful in differentiating one from the other.

As soon as Vikshepa is removed, the bliss of Savikalpa Samadhi manifests. This is Rasasvada. This is an obstacle for the attainment of the supreme bliss of Nirvikalpa Samadhi. The bliss of this Rasasvada is tantamount to the pleasure enjoyed by a cooly when he puts down a heavy load from his head, or the pleasure enjoyed by a man when he has killed a serpent which is guarding a vast hidden treasure. Only when he takes the treasure he enjoys the highest bliss. Even so, when the aspirant tastes the bliss of Nirvikalpa Samadhi, he has reached the zenith or culminating point. Killing of the serpent represents eradication of Vikshepa.

When meditation is practised, obstacles such as absence of right enquiry, impatience, laziness, inclination to enjoyment, absorption in sensual and impure thoughts come. Remove them through right enquiry and discrimination.

The Rajas and Tamas try their level best to re-enter the mental factory and take possession of their lost seats. They should be driven out by Viveka, Vichara and Vairagya (discrimination, enquiry of "Who am I ?" and dispassion). Impatience should be eradicated by practising patience. One should practise Sama, Dama and Uparati again and again.

Thoughts of Atman will remove impure thoughts (substitution method). Asana, Pranayama and light Sattvic diet will remove laziness.

18. A SYNOPTIC SURVEY OF DHYANA YOGA

What is Dharana ?

Dharana is concentration. It is fixing the mind on an external object or an internal point.

Concentration is purely a mental process. It needs an inward turning of the mind.

If you concentrate your mind on a point for 12 seconds, it is Dharana. Twelve such Dharanas will be a Dhyana (meditation). Twelve such Dhyanas will be Samadhi (superconsciousness).

Aids to Concentration

Cultivate attention; you will have good concentration.

A serene mind is fit for concentration. Keep the mind serene.

Be cheerful always. Then alone can you concentrate.

Be regular in your concentration. Sit in the same place, at the same time, 4 a.m.

Celibacy, Pranayama, reduction of wants and activities, dispassion, silence, discipline of the senses, Japa, control of anger, giving up the reading of novels, newspapers and visiting cinemas are all aids to concentration.

Japa (recitation of Lord's name) and Kirtan (singing of Lord's name and His glory) will develop concentration.

Stick to one centre when you concentrate.

Concentration demands patient and protracted practice.

Do not leave the practice even for a day. It is very difficult to rise up again.

How to Concentrate?

Silence the bubbling thoughts. Calm the surging emotions. Then alone will you be able to concentrate.

Concentrate on a concrete form in the beginning: on a flower, on the form of Lord Buddha, on any dream picture, on the effulgent light of the heart, on the picture of any saint, or your Ishta Devata.

Have 3 or 4 sittings: early morning, 8 a.m., 4 p.m. and 8 p.m.

Devotees concentrate on the heart, Raja Yogins on Trikuti (the seat of mind), Vedantins on Sahasrara or top of the head. Trikuti is the space between the eyebrows.

You can also concentrate on the tip of the nose, the navel or the Muladhara (below the last vertebra of the spinal column).

1. On Ishta Devata

Sit on any comfortable pose. Place a picture of your Ishta Devata in front of you. Look at the picture with steady gaze. Then close your eyes and visualise the picture in the centre of your heart or in the space between the eyebrows.

When the picture fades out in your mental vision, open the eyes and gaze at the picture again. Close your eyes after a few seconds and repeat the process.

2. For Christians

Devotees of Lord Jesus can concentrate on the picture of Lord Jesus or on the cross, in the same manner as stated above.

3. Gross Forms

Concentrate on a black dot on the wall, a candle flame, a bright star, the moon, on the picture of OM or any other object pleasant to you.

When you feel strain in your eyes, then close them for a minute and mentally visualise the object. When the mind runs again and again bring it back to the object of your concentration.

Concentration on the moon is beneficial to those of emotional temperament. Concentration on candle flame will give vision of Rishis and Devatas.

4. Subtle Methods

Concentrate on divine qualities such as love, mercy, compassion, or any other abstract idea such as infinity, omnipotence and omnipresence of the Lord, etc.

Read two or three pages of a book. Then close the book. Focus your attention carefully on the subject you have read. Abandon all other thoughts. Allow the mind to associate, classify, group, compare and combine the subject. You will get now a fund of knowledge and information on the subject. You will develop a good memory.

Lie on your bed in the open air and concentrate upon the blue expansive sky above. Your mind will expand immediately. You will be elevated. The blue sky will remind you of the infinite nature of the Self.

5. On Sounds

Sit on any comfortable pose. Close your eyes. Plug the ears with your index fingers or cotton plugs. Try to hear the Anahata sounds such as the music of the flute or violin, kettledrum, thunderstorm, chiming of bells, blowing of conch, humming of bees, etc. Hear only one kind of sound. Withdraw the mental rays from other objects and merge them in the sound you are trying to hear. You will get one-pointedness of mind. The mind can be controlled easily because it is enchanted by sweet notes.

Concentrate on the tick-tick sound of a watch.

Sit by the side of a river at a secluded spot. Concentrate your mind on the rushing sound of the river. You will hear the roaring of Om. This is very thrilling and inspiring

6. The Sufi Method

Place a mirror in front of you. Concentrate on the space between the eyebrows of your reflection in the mirror.

7. On Trikuti

The mind can be easily controlled by concentrating on the Trikuti, because it is the seat of the mind.

When there is deep concentration on Trikuti, you will experience great joy and spiritual intoxication. You will forget the body and the surroundings. All the Prana will be taken up to your head.

Gazing on a crystal or a Saligram induces concentration. You can concentrate on the breath in your nostrils (Soham sound). There is "So" during inhalation and "Ham" during exhalation.

General Hints

Do not concentrate when the mind is tired.

Do not wrestle with the mind when you concentrate.

When irrelevant thoughts enter the mind, be indifferent. They will pass away.

Do not drive them forcibly. They will persist and resist. It will tax your will. They will enter with redoubled force. But substitute divine thoughts. Evil thoughts will gradually fade out.

Be slow and steady in the practice of concentration.

Apply Brahmi-Amla oil to the head if there is much heat.

Take butter and sugar-candy. This will cool the system.

If you want to succeed in any walk of life, you must develop concentration. It is a source of spiritual strength. It is the master-key for opening the chamber of knowledge.

DHYANA (MEDITATION)

Meditation is an unbroken flow of knowledge of the object on which one meditates.

Meditation follows concentration. Concentration merges in meditation.

Meditation is the seventh step in the ladder of Yoga.

Concentration, meditation and Samadhi are internal Sadhanas.

When you practise concentration, meditation and Samadhi at a time, it is called Samyama.

Meditation is freeing the mind from all thoughts of sense-objects. The mind dwells on God alone during meditation.

Benefits of Meditation

If you meditate for half an hour daily, you will be able to face the battle of life with peace and spiritual strength.

Meditation kills all pain, suffering and sorrow.

Meditation is the most powerful mental and nervine tonic.

The divine energy freely flows off the Sadhaka during meditation and exercises a benign, soothing influence on the mind, nerves, sense organs and body.

Meditation is the mystic ladder which takes the Yogic student from earth to heaven.

Meditation is the key to unlock many of the secrets of life.

Meditation opens the door to intuitive knowledge and realms of eternal bliss.

During meditation the mind becomes calm, serene and steady. One idea occupies the mind.

Deep meditation cannot come in a day or a week or a month. You will have to struggle hard for a long time. Be patient. Be persevering. Be vigilant. Be diligent.

Cultivate burning dispassion, burning aspiration or an intense longing for Self-realisation. Gradually you will enter into deep meditation and Samadhi.

All doubts will be gradually cleared through meditation.

A mysterious inner voice will guide you. You will yourself feel the way to place your first step in the next rung of the Yogic ladder

How to Meditate?

Meditate regularly in the early morning between 4 and 6. The mind is calm and refreshed at that hour. The atmosphere also is calm. You will get good meditation.

Have a separate meditation room, or convert by means of screens a corner of a room into a meditation chamber. If there is much strain in your meditation, for a few days, reduce the duration of each sitting. Do light meditation.

Use your commonsense throughout your Sadhana. Do not go to extremes. Stick to the golden medium or the middle path.

Saguna Meditation

Mind wants a concrete object for meditation in the beginning.

Meditate in the beginning on a concrete form such as the image of your Ishta Devata, Lord Jesus, or Lord Buddha. This is Saguna meditation, or meditation on the form of the Lord with attributes.

Think of His attributes such as omnipotence, perfection, purity, freedom, when you meditate on His form.

Rotate your mind on His form from head to foot or from foot to head.

Meditation on Jesus

Place a picture of Jesus in front of you. Sit in your favourite meditative pose. Concentrate gently on the picture, with eyes open till you feel strain. Rotate the mind on his long hair, beautiful beard, round eyes, the cross on his chest and other limbs of the body, on the spiritual aura around the head, and so on.

Think of his divine attributes such as love, magnanimity, mercy and forbearance. Think of the various phases of his interesting life and the miracles he performed and the various extraordinary powers he possessed. Then close your eyes and try to visualise the picture. Repeat the same process again and again.

Meditation on Lord Hari

Place a picture of Lord Hari in front of you. Sit in a meditative posture. Concentrate gently on the picture. Rotate the mind on His feet, legs, yellow silken robes, golden garlands set with diamonds, Koustubha gem, etc. on his chest, then on the face, the ear-rings, the crown of the head, the discus on the right upper hand, the conch on the left upper hand, the mace on the right lower hand. Then close the eyes and try to visualise the picture in the same manner. Repeat the process again and again.

Devotees of Lord Buddha can meditate on his form in a similar way, in association with his particular attributes.

Meditation on Om

Have the picture of Om in front of you. Concentrate gently on this picture with open eyes. Associate the ideas of eternity, infinity, immortality, etc., when you think of Om. The humming of bees, the sweet notes of the nightingale, the seven notes of the scale in music—all sounds are emanations of Om only. Om is the essence of the Vedas. Imagine that Om is the bow, the mind is the arrow and Brahman or God is the target. Aim at the target with great care and then, like the arrow becoming one with the target, you will become one with God. You can also recite Om while meditating. The short accented Om burns all sins, the long accented gives Moksha, and the elongated bestows all psychic powers (Siddhis). He who chants and meditates upon this monosyllable (OM), meditates upon and chants all the scriptures of the world.

Abstract Meditations

Meditate on the effulgence in the sun, or the splendour in the moon, or the glory in the stars.

Meditate on the magnificence of the ocean and its infinite nature. Then compare the ocean to the infinite Brahman, and the waves, foams and icebergs to the various names and forms of the world. Identify yourself with the ocean. Become silent. Expand. Expand.

Meditate on the Himalayas. Imagine that the Ganga takes its origin in the icy regions of Gangotri, flows through

Rishikesh, Hardwar, Banaras, and then enters the Bay of Bengal near Gangasagar. The Himalayas, the Ganga and the sea: these three thoughts only should occupy your mind. First, take the mind to the icy regions of the Himalayas, then along the Ganga, and finally to the sea. Rotate the mind in this manner.

Gaze steadily on the formless air. Concentrate on the air. Meditate on the all-pervading nature of the air. This will lead to the realisation of the nameless and formless Brahman, the one, living Truth.

Watch the flow of breath. You will hear the sound "Soham", "So" during inhalation and "Ham" during exhalation. Soham means "I am He." The breath is reminding you of your identity with the Supreme Soul. You are unconsciously repeating Soham 21,600 times daily at the rate of 15 Sohams per minute. Associate the ideas of existence, Knowledge, Bliss, absolute purity, peace perfection, love, etc., along with Soham. Negate the body while repeating the Mantra and identify yourself with the Atman or the Supreme Soul.

Meditate on Nirguna Brahman or the Absolute. Think that there is a living, universal Power which underlies all names and forms. Associate the attributes of infinity, eternity, immortality, existence-consciousness-bliss absolute. In due course the attributes will merge in pure Nirguna meditation.

Experiences in Meditation

The feeling of rising up during meditation is a sign that you are going above body consciousness.

When you practise concentration and meditation, you are bound to get various Powers and Siddhis. Do not use these powers for gaining some material end. Do not misuse the powers. You will get a hopeless downfall.

Siddhis are obstacles in the path of Yoga. They are temptations. They will prevent you from entering into Samadhi or reaching the goal. Shun them ruthlessly and march direct to the goal.

There is really no such thing as a miracle. When you know the cause, the miracle becomes an ordinary event.

During meditation you will get rapture, ecstasy, thrill.

When you get a flash of illumination, do not be frightened. It will be a new experience of immense joy.

Do not be unnecessarily alarmed when you go above body-consciousness. Do not stop your Sadhana. The Lord will take care of you and guide you. Be bold. Do not look back. March on, Hero!

A flash is a glimpse of Truth. It is Ritambhara Prajna. This is not the whole experience. This is not the highest experience.

Reach the Bhuma or the Infinite. This is the acme or the final stage. You have reached the final destination. Meditation stops here.

You will hear various sorts of Anahata sounds, viz., bell, flute, lute, Veena, Mridanga and drum sounds, thunder, etc.

You will see brilliant lights in the space between the two eyebrows. They are like pin points, or like the sun, the moon or the stars. You will have vision of unity.

Sometimes you will behold coloured lights; green, blue, red, etc. They are due to the presence of different Tattvas at a particular time.

Prithvi or earth Tattva has yellow light; water Tattva white light; fire Tattva red light; air, smoky light or green light; Akasa, blue light. Ignore these lights and march forward.

Sometimes you will have visions of Rishis, sages, tutelary deity, Nitya Siddhas, astral entities, landscapes, mountains, blue sky, beautiful gardens.

Sometimes you may float in the air. Your astral body may get detached from the physical body. You will move about in the astral world.

You may go to Brahma Loka, the realm of Brahma or Hiranyagarbha.

Those who have entered the first degree of meditation will have a light body, sweetness of voice, beautiful complexion, clarity of mind and scanty urine and defaecation.

SAMADHI

What is Samadhi? Samadhi is superconscious state. It is union with God or the supreme Brahman.

The state of Samadhi is beyond description. There is no means or language to give expression to it.

You will have to experience this yourself through direct, intuitive cognition. Can you explain the taste of sugarcandy?

The state of Samadhi is all-bliss, joy and peace. This much only can be said. One has to feel this oneself.

In Samadhi the meditator loses his individuality and becomes identical with the Supreme Self. Just as camphor becomes identical with the fire, the meditator and the meditated become one.

Just as the river joins the ocean, the individual soul joins the Supreme Soul, the ocean of Absolute Consciousness.

This blissful divine experience arises when the ego and the mind are dissolved.

Samadhi is not like a stone-like inert state as many foolish persons imagine.

This is a magnificent experience of unity and oneness.

It is an experience wholly beyond the orbit of the senses. The seer and the sight become one.

In the state of Samadhi the aspirant is not conscious of any external or internal objects. There is no thinking, hearing, smelling or seeing.

Samadhi is the property of every human being.

Aids to Samadhi

Faith, power of concentration of mind, memory for contemplation, celibacy and discernment (Prajna) are the means for the attainment of Samadhi.

God's grace alone can take you to the realms of transcendental experience of Nirvikalpa Samadhi.

Jada and Chaitanya Samadhi

The Samadhi of the Hatha Yogi who buries himself is Jada Samadhi. It is like deep sleep. There is no transcendental, divine wisdom for him. The Samskaras are not burnt. He cannot have Moksha or final liberation.

In Chaitanya Samadhi there is perfect awareness. There is no rebirth. The Yogi attains liberation and divine wisdom.

Savikalpa Samadhi

There are two kinds of Samadhi viz., Savikalpa and Nirvikalpa.

Savikalpa Samadhi is also known as Samprajnata and Sabeeja Samadhi.

In Savikalpa Samadhi there is the Triputi or the triad: the knower, knowledge and the knowable.

Samprajnata or Savikalpa Samadhi is possible when there is Ekagrata or one-pointedness of mind.

There is only a partial inhibition of the mind.

The Samskaras or impressions are not burnt. Hence the name Sabeeja.

When the Yogi meditates on the Sattvic mind itself, devoid of Rajas and Tamas, he attains intense joy. So it is known as Sananda Samadhi or blissful Samadhi.

The Yogi feels "Aharn Asmi" or " I am", so, it is called Asmita Samadhi.

Nirvikalpa Samadhi

Nirvikalpa Samadhi is a condition of perfect awareness.

The knowledge and the knowable become one.

In Nirvikalpa Samadhi the Yogi sees without eyes, tastes without tongue, hears without ears, smells without nose and touches without skin.

This is described as follows: The blind man pierced the pearl; the fingerless put a thread into it; the neckless wore it and the tongueless praised it.

Nirvikalpa Samadhi is also known as Asamprajnata and Nirbeeja Samadhi.

There is complete inhibition of all mental functions. Hence it is called Asamprajnata Samadhi.

It can be attained only when there is perfect Nirodha or control of mind.

Here Samskaras are burnt in toto. Hence the name Nirbeeja.

Nirvikalpa Samadhi alone can destroy rebirth.

But, a mere glimpse of Truth cannot free you from birth and death.

You will have to be perfectly established in Nirvikalpa Samadhi. Then alone will the seed of rebirth be burnt in toto.

When the Yogi has reached the highest stage of Nirvikalpa Samadhi, the Yoga fire burns all the residue of his actions. He at once gets liberation in this very life. He attains immortality, the highest or transcendental wisdom and eternal bliss.

The only Sadhana for attaining Nirvikalpa Samadhi is Para Vairagya or supreme dispassion.

Here the Yogi completely disconnects himself from Prakriti and its effects.

The mind, intellect and the senses entirely cease to function.

There is neither sound nor touch nor form here.

All afflictions viz., ignorance, egoism, likes and dislikes, clinging to mundane life are destroyed now.

The Gunas, having fulfilled their objects of enjoyment, entirely cease to act now.

The Yogi has attained Kaivalya, or supreme Independence of freedom.

He has simultaneous knowledge or omniscience now.

The past and the future are blended into the present. Everything is 'now'. Everything is 'here!'

The Yogi has transcended time and space.

All sorrows have ceased; all miseries have disappeared; the seeds of actions are burnt; all doubts are dispelled. There is eternal freedom.

It is a state like the ocean without waves.

Chapter Two

THE ELIXIR OF BLISS

1. ASHTANGA YOGA

Practise first Ahimsa or non-injury,
Let this be in thought, word and deed;
Practise perfect truth and celibacy;
Truth alone triumphs but not falsehood.

Convert sex-energy into spiritual Ojas,
Never steal others' property,
Covet not others' wealth;
Be pure within and without.

Lead a life of contentment,
Practise Tapas to purify the heart,
And shine like the blazing fire;
Study the scriptures and roll the beads.

Surrender the fruits of actions unto the Lord,
Abandon agency and expectation of results;
Make your will one with the Cosmic Will,
Give up responsibilities and be at ease.

Sit harmonised with head, neck, trunk in a line,
Have God as your supreme goal;
Get mastery over the Pose Padma or Siddha,
Sit adamant, like that yonder rock.

Do not shake or scratch the body,
Body is a mould prepared by the mind,
If you shake the body the mind will be agitated,
Have a seat of cloth, tiger skin and Kusa grass.

Regulate the incoming and outgoing breath,
Practise Rechak, Kumbhak and Purak;

Retain not your breath beyond your capacity,
Purify thus the Nadis and steady the mind.

Now comes the withdrawal of the Indriyas;
This is Pratyahara or abstraction,
Which will check the outgoing senses
And keep them in their respective centres.

Fix the mind steadily on your point or Lakshya,
This is concentration which precedes meditation;
Allow the one thought of God to flow steadily,
This is meditation or divine contemplation.

Siddhis will manifest when there is concentration,
Shun them ruthlessly as they are obstacles;
Soar high in the realm of illimitable bliss,
Attain Kaivalya and achieve independence.

Samadhi will ensue after deep meditation
Samadhi is superconciousness that destroys Samskaras,
Samadhi will give you illumination and bliss,
Samadhi will free you from the round of births and deaths.

2. THE STEPS AND THE GOAL

Yama, Niyama, Asana, Pranayama
Prepare the Yogic student for concentration and meditation.
Concentration is the beginning of inner Yogic life,
Meditation is the middle.
Samadhi is the culmination.
Concentration is the key of all Yogas.
Meditation is the continuation of concentration.
Samadhi is the continuation of meditation.
Samadhi is the acme or perfection of Yoga.
Samadhi is the fruit of meditation
When you chant OM loudly
All other sounds are hushed and drowned in OM.
Even so when you raise the Brahmakara Vritti
All other sensual Vrittis perish.
They are fused in the one Brahmakara Vritti.

3. CONCENTRATION

Real Raja Yoga starts from concentration.
Fixing the mind on one point is concentration.
Concentration or Dharana merges in meditation (Dhyana)
Concentration is a portion of meditation.
Concentration ends in meditation.
And meditation ends in Samadhi.
It is difficult to say where Pratyahara ends
And concentration begins.
Where concentration ends
And meditation begins.
Concentration, meditation, Samadhi constitute Samyama.
Concentration for 20 seconds makes one meditation.
Twenty such meditations make one Samadhi.
This is for beginners.

4. THE POWER OF CONCENTRATION

If you focus the rays of the sun through a lens
They can burn cotton or piece of paper.
But the scattered rays cannot do this act.
If you want to talk to a man at a distance
You make a funnel of your hand and speak.
The sound waves are collected at one point
And then directed towards the man.
He can hear your speech very clearly.
The water is converted into steam
And the steam is converged at a point.
The Railway engine moves.
The steam in the cooking vessels moves the lid
                          and produces pat-pate sound.
All these are instances of concentrated waves.
Even so, if you collect the dissipated rays of the mind,
And focus them at a point,
You will have wonderful concentration.
The concentrated mind will serve as a potent searchlight,
To find out the treasures of the Soul
And attain the supreme wealth of the Atman.

Eternal bliss, immortality and perennial joy,
Therefore practise concentration and meditation regularly.

5. AIDS TO CONCENTRATION

Kumbhaka helps concentration
It checks the velocity of the mind
It makes the mind move in smaller circles
And ultimately curbs all its wanderings.
Trataka is a potent aid to concentration,
Fix the mind on the candle flame or a black dot
Or Sivalinga or Saligram.
Brahmacharya helps concentration.
Without Brahmacharya you cannot have definite progress,
Sattvic food is another aid to concentration,
Seclusion, Mouna, Satsanga, Asana, Japa,
Practice of Yama, Niyama, fasting,
Moderation in diet, non-mixing with persons,
Little talking, little exertion, little walking
Are all aids to concentration.

6. PATIENCE IN CONCENTRATION

An impatient man cannot practise concentration,
He gets up from his seat within a few seconds,
He gives up the practice within a week or month.
Concentration demands asinine patience.
It is very disgusting and tiring in the beginning,
As you have to take up the mental current upwards,
Like taking the Ganges water to Badri Narayan.
Later on it bestows infinite peace and bliss.
To dress a wound, clean the puss, is disgusting
In the beginning. For the first year medical student,
Later on, when he becomes a surgeon, F.R.C.S.
It is all intense pleasure for him to do operation daily.
He found M & B 693 times.
A doctor who found out a remedy for a certain disease
Made similar experiments C. D. 10,889 times.
A bird tried to empty the ocean with a blade of grass.

You must have patience like the bird and the doctor.
Then alone you will succeed in Yoga.

7. OBJECTS FOR CONCENTRATION

I

You can concentrate on a candle flame
Black dot on the wall, early morning or setting sun,
                             moon, stars,
"Bum sound of Ganges, Anahat sounds,
Any one of the Chakras in the body.
Saguna Murtis or Nirguna Brahman.
Abstract ideas as Bliss, peace, purity,
Perfection, freedom, independence,
Sounds of Mantras, Soham-breath in the nose,
Blue sky, all-pervading air or ether or light,
Effulgent light in the heart,
Sattvic, divine dream pictures,
Form of saints, Mahavakyas as "Tat Tvam Asi,"
OM symbol, significance of OM,
Form of your Guru and his divine attributes,
Or any thing your mind likes best.

II

Practise various sorts of concentration.
This will train or discipline your mind wonderfully.
Now concentrate on the Himalayas, a very great object.
Then concentrate on a mustard or a pin point.
Now concentrate on a distant object.
Then concentrate on a near object.
Then concentrate on a colour, sound, touch, smell or taste.
Then concentrate on the "tick-tick" of a watch.
Now concentrate on the virtue, mercy.
Now concentrate on the virtue, patience.
Now concentrate on the Sloka "Jyotishamapi Tat Joyti"
Then concentrate on "Satyam Jnanam Anantam".
Now concentrate on the Virat Purusha.
Then concentrate on Hiranyagarbha.

Now concentrate on the image of Lord Siva.
Then concentrate on "Aham Brahma Asmi" Mahavakya.

8. BENEFITS OF CONCENTRATION

It helps the scientists and Professors
To do great research work.
It helps the doctor and the lawyer
To do much work and earn more money,
It develops will power, memory,
Sharpens and brightens the intellect,
It bestows serenity or calmness of mind,
Inner spiritual strength, patience,
Great capacity to turn out tremendous work,
Alacrity, acumen, agility,
Beautiful complexion, sweet voice,
Brilliant eyes, powerful voice and speech,
Power to influence others and attract people,
Cheerfulness, joy, bliss of soul, supreme peace,
It removes restlessness, agitation of mind, laziness,
It makes you fearless and unattached
It helps you to attain God-Realisation.

9. MEDITATION

Dhyana is meditation
Dhyanam Nirvishayam Manah—
Meditation is freeing the mind from all objects,
And thoughts of sensual enjoyment.
If this is done, God-Realisation will come by itself.
God will enthrone in your heart immediately.
Meditation will come by itself without any effort.
If you bring a light in a dark cave
Which is filled with darkness for thousands of years,
The darkness will vanish at once by itself.
You need not strive hard to drive the darkness away.
If you attempt to put your hand in a pot,
Which is filled with various sorts of dust and dirt
You cannot.

Empty the dust and dirt,
You can put your hand inside the pot quite easily.
Even so if you empty the mind of its dirt and Vishayas
God will enter the mind in a twinkling of an eye.

II

Do not sit for meditation
When there is an urgent engagement.
The mind will be restless.
It will be ever thinking of the engagement only.
You will have no concentration.
Lead the divine life daily.
Express it in your daily life.
Then alone meditation will bear fruit.
Sit on the Ganges bank or in the temple.
You will have good meditation.
Repeat Guru Stotra, Santipatha or some prayers
Before you start meditation.
Be patient, be dispassionate, persevere.
Be bold, be wise, be pure.
You will attain success in meditation.
You will enter into Nirvikalpa Samadhi,
Wherein all ideas perish.

III

Salute Lord Ganesa and your Guru first.
Forget the past.
Old memories will trouble you during meditation.
Become indifferent; think of the object of meditation.
Control the emotions and impulses.
Be patient; do not try to get up soon
When you get pain in the legs.
Persevere, plod on, be courageous.
Sit and meditate in a solitary place.
Give up planning and building castles in the air.
Drive off sleepiness and Tandri by Kumbhaka and Kirtan.
Bring the mind in smaller circles first,
When it is fixed, do not disturb it.
Do not allow it to slip in the old grooves.

10. MEDITATE REGULARLY

Be contented, cheerful and serene:
Then alone you can practise meditation.
Meditation cannot arise in an agitated or restless mind.
Harbour not any grievance against anybody;
Excuse that man who speaks ill of you,
Pity him and say: "He is an ignorant, undeveloped soul."
Sometime coax and cajole the mind just as you do your child
Sometime mock and ridicule it and put it in shame,
Sometime curb it but use not violent methods:
Thus control the mind skilfully and tactfully—
Meditate regularly and reach the goal quickly.

11. FOUR KINDS OF MEDITATION

There are four kinds of Dhyana or meditation,
Viz., Sthoola (gross), Sookshma (subtle),
Sookshmatara (more subtle) and Sookshmatama
                                    (most subtle)
Savitarka and Nirvitarka are gross meditation.
Savichara and Nirvichara are subtle meditation.
Sananda is more subtle meditation.
Sasmita is the most subtle meditation.
Meditation on the form of Lord Vishnu with four hands,
Is gross meditation.
Meditation on the virtues is subtle meditation.
Meditation on the light is also subtle meditation.
Meditation on beauty, bliss, peace is more subtle meditation.
Meditation on the formless Brahman is most subtle meditation
Sthoola or gross meditation is concrete meditation.
Sookshma or subtle meditation is abstract meditation.

12. THE INVERSE PROCESS

Meditate on the Karana:
Negate the Karya.
The objects are the Karya
Of the five elements which are the Karana.
The five elements are the Karya

Of Prakriti which is the Karana.
Like this go from the gross to the subtle.
This will lead you to Brahman,
The Causeless Cause of everything.
This is a potent method of meditation.

13. VEDANTIC ENQUIRY OF VICHARA
(Laya Chintana)

This body is made up of five elements.
Now imagine, meditate and feel:
The earth-portion of this body
Gets dissolved into the Prithvi Tattva
The watery portion into the Apas Tattva
The fiery portion into the Tejas Tattva
The airy portion into the Vayu Tattva
The ethereal portion into the Akasa Tattva.
The mind, Chitta, intellect and Ahamkara
Get dissolved into the Mula Prakriti.
Now what remains?
The residual (Sesha) is your own Atman
The All-pervading, Immortal Soul
That Thou Art, O Ram!
Tat Tvam Asi!
Feel this, realise this
And be free!

14. MEDITATION ON VIRTUES

Courage, temperance, justice,
Truthfulness, non-violence, purity, mercy,
Humility, tolerance, forbearance,
Are all important virtues.
Benevolence, charity, generosity,
Are other virtues.
Meditate constantly on these virtues.
Think of the benefit of possessing these virtues.
Eradicate evil qualities.
You will develop the above virtues,

Meditate on Atman, the source for everything.
Meditate on the Lord,
Who possesses all these virtues,
Who has Ananta Kalyana Gunas,
You will develop all virtues.

15. DHYANA YOGA (SAGUNA)

Get steadiness in pose,
Keep the head, neck and trunk in a line;
Do not shake the body.
Remain like a statue.
By practice sit for three hours.
Meditate in Brahmamuhurta;
Close the eyes and meditate,
In the Trikuti or the heart;
Yogis concentrate in the Trikuti,
Bhaktas select the heart;
Visualise the picture of the Lord,
Rotate the mind from feet to head.
Face East or North,
Sit in Padma or Siddhasana;
You can have Sukha Asana too;
Repeat some prayers to begin with.
Have two or three sittings daily,
Have rigorous Sadhana in winter,
Meditation follows concentration,
Samadhi follows meditation.
Repeat the Name of the Lord,
Think of His attributes too;
Remember His Leelas also,
This will strengthen meditation.
Bring the mind again and again,
To the point, centre or Lakshya;
Be patient in your practice,
Then only you will attain success.
Meditation shuts worldly thoughts,
Meditation increases Sattva,

Meditation gives good health,
Meditation makes you divine.
Meditation kills pains and sorrows,
Meditation destroys rebirths,
Meditation gives peace and bliss;
Therefore meditate regularly.

16. DHYANA YOGA (NIRGUNA)

This is meditation on Brahman,
Who is non-dual and attributeless,
Who is self-luminous and indivisible,
Who is pure and changeless.
Practise first the Neti Neti doctrine,
Negate the illusory Upadhis,
Sublate the Prana, mind and body,
Throw away the sheaths as non-self.
Just as you take the pith from the grass,
The butter from the milk,
Take the essence of Brahman,
Through the churning of meditation.
Enquire 'Who am I'?
Meditate 'I am Sat-Chit-Ananda',
Feel 'I am Sakshi'
Identify with the Self.
Feel 'I am distinct from the bodies,
I am distinct from the sheaths,
I am witness of the three states,
I am Eternal Changeless Atman'
Repeat mentally OM OM OM,
With Bhava and feeling,
Or associate 'So' with inhalation,
And 'Hum' with exhalation.
Meditate on the Maha Vakya,
'Aham Brahma Asmi'
Or 'Sivoham' formula,
And enter into Nirvikalpa Samadhi.
Assert, recognise, realise,

'I am Light of lights, OM OM OM'
'I am Immortal Self, OM OM OM'
'I am Consciousness, OM OM OM'
Feel 'I am not actor',
'I am not enjoyer',
'I am Akarta, Abhokta',
'I am Asanga, Unattached.'
Repeat 'Soham Sivoham,
Aham Brahmasmi,
Sat-Chit-Ananda
Svaroopoham.'
'Hamsa Soham, Soham Hamsa,
Hamsa Soham, Soham Hamsa,
Hamsa Soham, Soham Hamsa,
Hamsa Soham, Soham Hamsa,'
'Brahmaivaham, Brahmaivaham,
Brahmaivaham, Brahmoham;'
Sivaivaham, Sivaivaham,
Sivaivaham, Sivoham.

17. MEDITATE ON THE LORD

Meditate on the Lord, the Inner Ruler,
The Indweller of your heart,
The lotus of your heart will blossom.
The sun of wisdom will shine,
The darkness of the heart will end,
The five Kleshas will be annihilated,
The three fires will be extinguished.
Sins and Samskaras will be burnt.
Vasanas and cravings will be fried.

18. MEDITATE ON THE ETERNAL

Meditate on the Eternal, free from pain,
From stain, from disease, from fear and delusion,
All-filling, pure, far yet near,
The birth place of five elements,
The final goal of Yogins and sages,

The source for mind, senses and the Vedas,
The place where silence reigns supreme,
Where there is immortal bliss beyond thought,
The supreme glorious splendour,
Where thought is dead,
The all-filling supreme Peace,
Where there is neither noise nor fight.

19. OBJECTS OF MEDITATION

Even Vedantic students have
The ideas of all-pervading ether
And Jyoti for their meditation in the beginning.
They get help from the external elements.
The Bhaktas cultivate one of the five Bhavas:
Santa, Dasya, Sakhya, Vatsalya and Madhurya,
And meditate on their object of Love.

20. OBSTACLES IN MEDITATION

I

Vishayasakti or attachment to objects,
Dullness of intellect or understanding,
Kutarka or ill-directed argument
Leading to misinterpretation of texts,
Vipareeta Bhavana or clinging obstinately
To the belief that Atman is susceptible,
To suffering, grief and enjoying happiness,
Are the four chief obstacles in meditation.
Any one of these is quite sufficient
To interfere with the attainment of real knowledge.
Therefore, cultivate Vairagya or dispassion.
Sharpen the intellect and give up
Kutarka and Vipareeta Bhavana
Identify yourself with the pure Atman,
You will soon attain knowledge of the Self.

II

The mind does two things
It ceaselessly thinks of sensual objects.

When it is tired of thinking of objects.
It goes to sleep and rests in Moola Avidya.
If sleep or Laya tries to overpower you during meditation
Awaken the mind, be on the alert.
If the mind is distracted on account of Vikshepa,
Calm it, render it serene.
If there is attachment to any object,
Wean the mind, make it unattached.
Again and again think of Brahman,
Start the Brahmachintana vigorously,
Abandon the bliss of Savikalpa Samadhi also.
It is also a hindrance to the highest realisation.
When the mind has become perfectly calm
Do not disturb it even a bit,
Continue the meditation vigorously.
You will soon enter into Nirvikalpa Samadhi,
And realise the supreme Universal bliss.

21. BE VIGILANT

If you are careless and non-vigilant,
If you are irregular in meditation,
If you yield even a bit to sensual pleasure,
The mind will continue to go downward
Like a ball dropped upon a flight of stairs.
When sedge is displaced on the surface of a lake
It closes in again at once.
Even so, Maya closes in even upon a wise man,
If he stops his meditation and Sadhana even for a short time.
Therefore be careful, be alert,
Be regular in your meditation.

22. DISCERN AND DISCRIMINATE

When the mind is sluggish or torpid, sleepy,
Rouse it by Kirtan, Japa, prayer, Pranayama,
Sarvanga, Sirshasana and long OM chanting.
When it is distracted,
Make it steady, one-pointed and calm

Through perseverance, dispassion,
Recourse to solitude, Japa, Trataka, Mouna or silence.
When it becomes attached,
Get it detached through dispassion,
Enquiry, vigilance, Dosha-drishti,
Or Finding out the defects of sensual life.
And Mithya-drishti, i.e. feeling that everything is unreal
When it is controlled,
Do not disturb it any more.

When you enjoy the bliss of Savikalpa Samadhi (Rasasvada)

23. MEDITATION AND KNOWLEDGE

Meditation is the means,
Knowledge is the end,
Meditation is the process,
Knowledge is the culmination.
In meditation there is struggle, striving of effort,
In knowledge there is no striving,
So long as there is meditation,
The meditator is only an aspirant.
When meditation ceases and the goal is reached,
The meditator becomes the knower of Truth,
All meditator and effort cease.
He is a Jeevanmukta or a liberated sage.
When you try to behold a tree,
There is an effort in the beginning of the perception.
Later on it becomes a continuous stream of
                            consciousness of the tree
So is knowledge of Brahman.
In the beginning there is effort.
Later on the aspirant merges in the object of meditation.
There is no further struggle.

24. SAMADHI

Samadhi is blissful union,
The Jiva unites with Brahman;
The third eye is opened,

The Indriyas are restrained,
The bubbling mind is stilled,
Names and forms vanish,
Brahman alone shines.
Vasanas he annihilates,
Thoughts he controls,
Cravings he crushes,
Attachments he cuts,
Egoism he kills,
Likes and dislikes he eradicates,
Knowledge of Self he attains.
The divine Nectar he now drinks,
Immortal he becomes,
In the Self he rejoices,
The Self he beholds everywhere,
I-less, griefless he becomes,
As a beacon-light he shines,
And joy he radiates to all.

25. SAMSKARA SESHA

Samskara means impressions of actions.
Sesha means remainder.
Samskara Sesha means remainder of impressions.
Savikalpa Samadhi of a Raja Yogin,
Who practises Savitarka, Savichara,
Nirvitarka, Nirvichara, Sananda,
Sasmita Samadhis, leaves the impressions
Of Vichara feeling of bliss,
And the feeling of "Aham Asmi" or "I exist."
This is called Samskara Sesha.
This corresponds to the Lesha Avidya of sages.
Even after one attains Jeevanmukti
He experiences a trace of Avidya.
On account of this he moves about,
Takes bath, answers calls of nature
And takes food and drinks.
The impression of Lesha Avidya is like that

Of the garlic smell which the pot emanates
Even after it is washed several times.

26. MIND FUSES IN SAMADHI

Camphor melts in the fire,
And assumes the form of fire;
When salt is dissolved in water,
It is no longer perceived separately;
The water alone remains.
Even so the mind that has assumed
The form of Brahman, which is secondless,
Is no longer perceived.
Brahman alone remains in its pristine glory.

27. NIRVIKALPA SAMADHI

In Nirvikalpa Samadhi
There is no ego-consciousness.
Ego and mind melt and fuse in Brahman.
The Triputi or the distinction of
Knower, knowledge and the object of knowing,
Vanishes in toto.
The pure mind assumes the form of Brahman.
This is known as Asamprajnata Samadhi,
Niralamba or Nirbija Samadhi.
There is no prop for the mind in this Samadhi,
Brahman rests in its own glory.
The Samskaras are fried in toto.
Savikalpa Samadhi deepens into Nirvikalpa Samadhi There
is no idea of any kind in Nirvikalpa Samadhi.
It is thoughtless Absolute Consciousness.

II

Nirvikalpa means that in which
There is no Vikalpa.
That which is not associated
With any idea is Nirvikalpa.
In Nirvikalpa Samadhi there is no thought,
No imagination, no functioning of mind or intellect.

All Vrittis totally cease.
There is only Pure Consciousness or Awareness.
All the Samskaras and Vasanas are fried in toto.
Egoism is burnt to ashes
The world of passion which is very charming
For the passionate worldlings
Is reduced to ashes.
All names and forms are bunt up.
Asti-Bhati-Priya only remains.
Asti-Bhati-Priya is Sat-Chit-Anada.
That which ever exists is Asti;
That which shines is Bhati;
This is absolute consciousness;
That which gives happiness is Priya.
This is unalloyed, Immortal Bliss, Ananda.
In Nirvikalpa Samadhi the mind
Is freed from distraction, attachments,
Torpidity and all other defects.
It rests unmoved like the flame of a lamp
Sheltered from the wind.

III

Nirvikalpa Samadhi is beyond all expressions.
All sense of duality is obliterated.
There is pure or Absolute Consciousness.
There is full illumination.
There is neither craving nor egoism.
The bliss of the sage is unending.
He is united with the Infinite,
He is free, perfect, independent.
He is freed from pain, sorrow and illusion.
He is an Apta Kama.
All his desires are gratified.
He has attained the state of Supreme Peace.

28. MYSTICISM

Mysticism is intuitionalism.
Mysticism is transcendentalism.

Mysticism is Aparoksha Anubhuti.
Mysticism is direct Self-realisation.
Mysticism is Anubhava Advaita.
Mysticism is spiritual, intuitive experience,
Which is beyond the reach of intellect.
Mysticism is Nirvikalpa Samadhi.
Mysticism is direct Communion with God.
Mystic is one who is versed in mysticism.

29. ALL IS AKHANDA EKARASA SVAROOPA

Para Brahman is Akhanda Ekarasa Svaroopa.
Guru is Akhanda Ekarasa Svaroopa.
The disciple is also Akhanda Ekarasa Svaroopa.
The Jiva is Akhanda Ekarasa Svaroopa.
The Sakshi is Akhanda Ekarasa Svaroopa.
Fire is Akhanda Ekarasa Svaroopa.
Water is Akhanda Ekarasa Svaroopa.
Air is Akhanda Ekarasa Svaroopa.
Akasa is Akhanda Ekarasa Svaroopa.
Mind is Akhanda Ekarasa Svaroopa.
Intellect is Akhanda Ekarasa Svaroopa.
The eye is Akhanda Ekarasa Svaroopa.
This world is Akhanda Ekarasa Svaroopa.
All is Akhanda Ekarasa Svaroopa.

30. MERGING OR FUSING

When you have realised Oneness,
When you behold the One Brahman everywhere,
Can there be a "here" or "there",
"This" or "That", "I", "He" or "You"?
Can there be "one" or "two" or "three"?
One homogeneous blissful essence alone exists.
There is only the Bhuma or the Infinite.
All dualities, distinctions, differences melt.
The seer and the seen become one,
The meditator and the meditated fuse.
The thinker and the thought blend.

The knower and the knowable merge.
It is a transcendental Experience Whole.
Of fullness, perfection, freedom and perennial joy.

31. SPIRITUAL EXPERIENCES

More and more dispassion and discrimination,
More and more yearning for liberation,
Peace, cheerfulness, contentment,
Fearlessness, unruffled state of mind,
Lustre in the eyes, good smell from the body,
Beautiful complexion, sweet, powerful voice,
Passing of little urine and excretion,
Wonderful health, vim, vigour and vitality,
Freedom from disease, laziness and depression,
Lightness of body, alertness of mind,
Powerful Jatharagni or digestive fire,
Eagerness to sit and meditate for a long time.
Aversion to worldly talks and company of worldlings, Feeling of the presence of God everywhere.
Love for all creatures,
Feeling that all forms are of the Lord.
That the world is Lord Himself.
Absence of Ghrina or dislike to any creature,
Even to those who despise and insult you,
Strength of mind to bear insult and injury,
To meet dangers and calamities,
Are some of the preliminary spiritual experiences.
These indicate that you are steadily advancing
In the spiritual path.

II

Balls of white lights, coloured lights,
Sun, stars, during meditation
Divya Gandha, Divya taste,
Vision of the Lord in the dream,
Extraordinary, superhuman experiences,
Vision of the Lord in the human form,
Sometime in the form of a Brahmin,

Old men, leper, outcaste in rags,
Talking to the Lord,
Are the preliminary spiritual experiences.
Then comes cosmic consciousness or Savikalpa Samadhi,
Which Arjuna experienced.
Eventually the aspirant enters
Into Nirvikalpa Samadhi,
Wherein there in neither seer nor seen,
Wherein one sees nothing, hears nothing,
He becomes one with the Eternal

32. I DRINK THE NECTAR

My Sat-Guru gave me a sword of wisdom.
He united me with the absolute.
He showed me the way to wipe my Karmas.
He removed many pitfalls and snares.
I realised the Supreme State of Changeless joy.
Wherein the seer, seen and sight are lost
I live in perfection everywhere.
I have nothing more to learn.
The disease of birth has left me.
I lost myself and became the mass of bliss.
I drink the nectar of Immortality,
Which is sweeter than all syrups.

33. SPEECHLESS ZONE

In the perfect nameless, formless Void,
In the unlimited expanse of bliss,
In the region of matterless, mindless joy,
In the realm of timeless, spaceless stillness,
In the Infinite Zone of speechless, thoughtless peace,
In the transcendental abode of sweet Harmony,
I united with the Supreme Effulgence.
The thought that we are one or two vanished.
I crossed the sea of birth for ever.
This is all due to the grace of the Lord,

Who danced in Brindawan with rhythmic jingle,
Who raised Govardhan as umbrella for the cowherds.

34. THAT EXALTED STATE

I searched God in the caves of the Himalayas,
In the pilgrim-centres, in river banks.
But I myself am Brahman, God of gods now!
I had once intense love for my sweet home;
Native village, district, and province.
But I am now the home of all worlds,
East and West, North and South,
Greece and India, Australia and France,
China and Russia have become one.
I loved Tamil once;
But I am "OM" now,
The source of all languages.
I had once great love for my body;
But now I have realised "All bodies are mine,"
Once one hundred years was too big for me;
But I now abide in Eternity;
No time-piece, no calendar is necessary now.
Once five thousand miles was a great distance for me.
But now I feel "I am Infinity."
Time, space have vanished.
I have neither home nor house, address nor name!

35. I LIVE IN SILENCE!

The world may call me good or abuse me,
I do not care now for criticism of the world.
Why should I? When my abode is transcendental!
I am now above good and evil; censure and praise.
I have no connection with body and mind.
I have neither hope, nor fear.
What have I to do with this world?
I am now swimming in the ocean of Brahmic bliss.
I do not want anybody's favour or recommendation.
I do not wish to interview anybody.

I care not for anybody's company or help.
I live in silence enjoy silence. I am silence!
Chelas! Chelas!! And all!!
Friends! Leave me now please!
Goodbye!

36. BLISSFUL AM I NOW

Home have I left; the world have I abandoned.
All my mundane desires I have relinquished.
The shallow, hollow nature of this world I have understood.
The worthlessness of all objects I realised.
Lust I have left, anger, pride I have given up.
Craving, longing for objects I overpowered.
I sat on the bank of the Ganga in the Himalayas.
I reflected, I contemplated deeply on Brahman,
Ignorance vanished;
My heart is healed.
All Trishnas were ousted from my heart.
All within is purity and peace,
Serene am I now; knowing the peace of the Eternal;
Blissful am I now; realising my essential nature.

37. MY HEART IS BRIMFUL OF JOY!

The three heart-knots are cut;
All ties have been severed.
All bonds have been broken
The three fires have been extinguished.
The five afflictions have been burnt
Old ignorance has vanished.
Maya is hiding herself in shame.
Poverty, nescience, disease have disappeared.
I am floating in the ocean of joy.
I am light, bliss, peace and harmony.
I have realised the Bhuma, the Great Bliss.
All darkness has been dispelled.
The world has melted in me.

I am a mass of bliss and wisdom.
My heart is brimful of joy and bliss.

38. WELCOME, DISEASE! WELCOME!!

Welcome disease! Welcome pain!
Welcome microbes! Welcome death!
Welcome malaria! Welcome pyorrhoea!
Welcome cholera! Welcome typhoid!
Welcome appendicitis! Welcome!! Welcome!!
I am not afraid of you all
Thou art my own manifestation.
The cataract of illusion has vanished;
I behold the light and Truth everywhere.
You are all my beloved guests in the body.
Health and disease are two ripples.
In the ocean of Bliss of Self.
Pain also is Pleasure for me!

39. I AM FULL NOW

I know the secret of Brahma Vidya.
I have realised my essential nature,
Maya is hiding herself,
She cannot show me Her face.
She is shy to appear before me.
Where shall I go now?
When I am all-pervading and infinite,
What shall I desire now?
What shall I take?
What shall I renounce?
What work shall I do now?
What is there to achieve?
What shall I seek?
When I am now an Aptakama,
When I possess the whole,
When all my desires are satisfied,
By the experience whole,
When I am full, Poornam;

What shall I read now,
When I am a man of wisdom, Chidghana?
To whom shall I deliver lecture
When I alone exist ?

40. THE LITTLE 'I' FUSED!

I sat alone on a block of stone
On the bank of the Ganges, of Bhagirathi.
Mother Ganga blessed me!
I meditated on OM and its meaning,
The Word that is the symbol of Brahman.
The little personality was lost.
The mortal limit of the Self was loosened!
But there was infinite extension,
I entered into the Nameless beyond.
I realised the quintessential unity of bliss.
No words can describe the thrill of joy,
The magnanimous mystic experience,
The supremest and divinest height of felicity;
The little 'I' fused into the incandescent brilliance.
Two became one now,
It was all Tejomaya Ananda,
One mass of transcendental Light-Bliss.

41. SAMADHI

I did Japa of OM.
I chanted OM, sang OM.
I meditated on OM.
The individuality slowly dissolved.
It faded away into the Infinite Being.
The loss of personality is no extinction.
It is the only true, whole, eternal life.
It is the Bhuma experience,
This exalted state is utterly beyond words.
It is not a confused state.
It is a state of ineffable bliss and joy.
It is the clearest of the clearest.

It is the surest of the surest.
It is like the apple in the palm of the hand.
Death here is a ridiculous impossibility.
Immortal elixir flows here perennially.
Wisdom shines in profound effulgence.
Perfect peace reigns supreme!

42. I HAVE BECOME THAT

The Maya-made world has vanished now!
Mind has totally perished.
The ego has been entirely powdered.
The water-tight compartments have been broken down.
Names and forms have disappeared.
All distinctions and differences have melted.
Old Jivahood has entirely fused;
The flood of Truth, Wisdom and Bliss
Has entered everywhere in abundance.
Brahman alone shines everywhere.
One homogeneous Joy essence pervades everywhere.
I have become That. I have become That!
Sivoham! Sivoham!! Sivoham!!!

43. I FOUND HIM OUT

I wandered, searched
And then I found Him out at last—
In the silence of the mind.
He is the wonder of wonders;
He is the nectar that never satiates,
He is knowledge's End,
He is the great primal Being.
He is the sweet celestial honey
That destroys old age and death,
He is the endless primeval light,
He is the medicine sweet
That confers Immortality.
I call Him 'a Mass of Sweetness',
I call Him 'the Ocean of Bliss',

I call Him 'the Old Man of the Upanishads',
I call Him 'the Silent sleeper in the Sea'

44. MYSTERIOUS EXPERIENCE

Brahman or the Eternal is far sweeter than honey,
Jam, sugar candy, Rasagullah or Laddu.
I meditated on Brahman the Immutable.
I attained the stage that transcends finite.
True light shone in me.
Avidya or ignorance vanished in toto.
The doors were totally shut;
The senses were withdrawn;
Breath and mind merged in their source.
I became one with the Supreme Light.
A mysterious experience beyond speech indeed.
Sivoham Sivoham Sivoham Soham.
Sat-Chit-Ananda Svaroopoham.

45. THE GREAT BHUMA EXPERIENCE

I merged myself in great unending joy,
I swam in the ocean of immortal bliss.
I floated in the sea of Infinite Peace.
Ego melted, thoughts subsided,
Intellect ceased functioning,
The senses were absorbed.
I remained unawakened to the world.
I saw myself everywhere.
It was a homogeneous experience.
There was neither within nor without;
There was neither "this" nor "that";
There was neither "here" nor "there";
There was neither "he", "you" or "I" or "she",
There was neither time nor space;
There was neither subject nor object;
There was neither knower nor knowable nor knowledge;
There was neither seer nor seen nor sight;
How can one describe this transcendental experience?

Language is finite, words are impotent,
Realise this yourself and be free!

46. SONG OF OM

OM OM OM OM OM OM OM
OM OM OM OM OM OM OM
OM is the symbol of Brahman.
OM is the Pranava of Vedas.
OM is the Source of all languages.
I sing OM, I chant OM.
I meditate on OM.
I do Japa of OM
Celestial music of sweet OM.
Vibrates in my heart.
Divine rapture of eternal OM
Inspires and elevates me,
And opens the portals of oneness within.

Chapter Three

FORMULAS FOR MEDITATION

1. I AM LIFE ETERNAL

I am That I am.
I am absolute consciousness.
I am all joy.
I am all Bliss.
I am al! intelligence.
I am life Eternal.
I am Infinity, Eternity, Immortality.
I am Truth, Wisdom and Light.

2. VEDANTIC MEDITATION

I am ageless
I am birthless
I am deathless
I am timeless
I am spaceless
I am causeless
I am formless
I am attributeless
I am fearless
I am changeless
I am nameless

3. I AM THE SOURCE

I am the Source for everything,
I am beginningless,
I am endless,
I am the Root for everything,

I am present everywhere,
I am the very Source of power and energy,

I am one, complete whole, perfect,
I am formless, changeless, indivisible,
I am the Law, the way, the life,
I am the source for life,
I am the vital principle,
I am wisdom, existence and bliss.

4. I AM THE ALL

1 am the Immortal Essence
I am the Infinite
Worlds are in me
I am the soul of all beings.
I am timeless and spaceless
I am beginningless and endless
I am immutable
I am the all
I am All in All
I am the one and the many.

5. I AM EXISTENCE

I am the All
I am All in All
I pervade and permeate all

6. FORMULAS FOR MEDITATION

I am that I am
I am life universal
I am Soul universal
I have neither defeat
Nor failure nor loss
For I am the Eternal
Besides me there is none else.
Universes may appear and disappear
Suns may appear and vanish

I always remain
I am Existence Absolute.

7. VEDANTIC MEDITATION—II

I am the Sat-Chit-Ananda Brahman.	OM OM OM
I am Nirakara Para-Brahman.	OM OM OM
I am Advaita Para-Brahman.	OM OM OM
I am Akhanda Paripoorna Brahman.	OM OM OM
I am Nitya, Suddha, Siddha, Buddha	OM OM OM
and Mukta Brahman.	OM OM OM
I am Sat-Chit-Ananda Svaroopa	
(Satchidananda Svaroopoham)	OM OM OM
I am Bhumananda Svaroopa	
(Bhumananda Svaroopoham)	OM OM OM
I am Jyotih Svaroopa	
(Jyotih Svaroopoham)	OM OM OM
I am Santi Svaroopa	
(Santi Svaroopoham)	OM OM OM
I am Nitya-Suddha Svaroopa	
(Nitya-Suddha Svaroopoham)	OM OM OM
I am Nitya Bodha Svaroopa	
(Nitya Bodha Svaroopoham)	OM OM OM
I am Nitya-Mukta Svaroopa	
(Nitya-Mukta Svaroopoham)	OM OM OM
I am Nitya-Tripti Svaroopa	
(Nitya-Tripti Svaroopoham)	OM OM OM
I am NityaVijnana Svaroopa	
(Nitya-Vijnana Svaroopoham)	OM OM OM
I am Nitya-Chaitanya Svaroopa	
(Nitya-Chaitanya Svaroopoham)	OM OM OM
I am the Atman of all	OM OM OM
I am the all	OM OM OM
I am the support of all	OM OM OM
I am the transcendent.	OM OM OM
I am the Brahman without caste,	OM OM OM
creed or colour.	OM OM OM
I am Nitya-Nishkala Brahman	OM OM OM

I am Nirmala and Nishkriya Brahman   OM OM OM
I am Akhanda-Ekarasa-Chinmatra Brahman
(Akhandaikarasa Chinmatroham)   OM OM OM
I am Nirvisesha Chinmatra Brahman.
(Nirvisesha Chinmatroham)   OM OM OM
I am Kevala Chinmatra Brahman
                 (Kevala Chinmatroham)   OM OM OM
I am Kevala-Sat-Matra Brahman (Kevala
                        Sanmatroham)   OM OM OM
I am Prajnana-ghana Brahman   OM OM OM
I am Vijnana-ghana Brahman   OM OM OM
I am Chit-ghana Brahman   OM OM OM
I am Ananda-ghana Brahman   OM OM OM
I am Chinmaya Brahman   OM OM OM
I am Anandamaya Brahman   OM OM OM
I am Jyotirmaya Brahman   OM OM OM
I am Tejomaya Brahman   OM OM OM
I am Nirakara, Nirguna, Nirvisesha Brahman   OM OM OM
I am Nirupadika, Nishkala Brahman   OM OM OM
I am Nirbhaya, Niravayava Brahman   OM OM OM
I am verily that Brahman, the One without
       a second which is very, very subtle,
       which illumines all things and which
       is eternal, pure and immovable.   OM OM OM
I am Satyam-Jnanam-Anantam Brahman.   OM OM OM
I am Anadi-Ananta Brahman.   OM OM OM
I am Amrita-Avinasi Brahman.   OM OM OM
I am Adhishthana and Aparichhinna
                         Brahman   OM OM OM
I am Mayatita Brahman.   OM OM OM
I am Dvandvatita Brahman.   OM OM OM
I am Trigunatita Brahman.   OM OM OM
I am Bhavatita Brahman.   OM OM OM
I am Nada Bindu Kalatita Brahman.   OM OM OM
I am Avyakta, Anusuta Brahman.   OM OM OM
I am Akasavat, Nitya Brahman.   OM OM OM

I am Desa-Kala-Vivarjita, Gagana
Sadrisha, Niralamba Brahman.   OM OM OM
I am Santa, Ajara, Amrita, Abhaya,
                 Para Brahman.   OM OM OM
I am Divya, Amurta, Aprana,
                 Amana Brahman.   OM OM OM
I am Sasvata, Svatantra, Kutashtha
                 Brahman.   OM OM OM
I am Asanga Brahman (Asangoham)   OM OM OM
I am Niranjana Brahman (Niranjanoham)   OM OM OM
I am Kutastha Brahman (Kutasthoham)   OM OM OM
I am Kevala Brahman (Kevaloham)   OM OM OM
I am the Source.   OM OM OM
I am the Supreme.   OM OM OM
I am Siva.   OM OM OM
I am He.   OM OM OM
I am Chaitanya.   OM OM OM
I am Sakshi.   OM OM OM
I am Drashta and Upadrashta.   OM OM OM
I am the Vetta.   OM OM OM
I am without the number two.   OM OM OM
I am Akhanda Chidakasa Brahman.   OM OM OM
I am Adhishthana Brahman.   OM OM OM
I am Avyaya Akshara Brahman.   OM OM OM
I am Nirmala Brahman.   OM OM OM
I am Vijnana Vigraha Brahman.   OM OM OM
I am Atindriya Brahman (Atindriyoham).   OM OM OM
I am Niramaya Brahman.   OM OM OM
I am Niravarana Brahman.   OM OM OM
I am Atisukshma Brahman.   OM OM OM
I am Nirdvandva Brahman.   OM OM OM
I am Nitya Nirupadhika Niratisaya
                 Ananda Brahman.   OM OM OM
I am Nirlipta Brahman.   OM OM OM
I am Asabda, Arupa and Agandha
                 Brahman.   OM OM OM
I am Nischala Brahman   OM OM OM

I am Avangmanogochara Brahman.   OM OM OM
I am Nirdosha Nirvikalpa Brahman.   OM OM OM
I am Anirdeshya, Adrishya Brahman.   OM OM OM
I am Kalatita, Desatita Brahman.   OM OM OM
I am Amala, Vimala, Nirmala Brahman.   OM OM OM
I am Achintya and Avyavahara. Brahman.   OM OM OM
I am equal in all (Samam).   OM OM OM
I am Purushottama.   OM OM OM
I am Isha.   OM OM OM
I am the Excellent.   OM OM OM
I am Siva.   OM OM OM
I am without language.   OM OM OM
I am without the "NO."   OM OM OM
I have no place to travel.   OM OM OM
I am within the within.   OM OM OM
I am the manifested Brahman.   OM OM OM
I am the unmanifested Brahman.   OM OM OM
I am the immanent Brahman.   OM OM OM
I am the transcendental, Trigunatita,
                Ananta-Brahman.   OM OM OM
I am Karana Brahman.   OM OM OM
I am Karya Brahman.   OM OM OM
I am the All.   OM OM OM
I am the All in All.   OM OM OM
I am the One in All.   OM OM OM
I am the All in One.   OM OM OM
I am the Many.   OM OM OM
I am ever waking when all
          living beings sleep at night.   OM OM OM
I shine even during the Cosmic Pralaya.   OM OM OM
I am the ancient One.   OM OM OM
I am alone.   OM OM OM
I am Single.   OM OM OM
I see now without eyes.   OM OM OM
I hear now without ears.   OM OM OM
I taste now without tongue.   OM OM OM
I feel now without skin.   OM OM OM

I smell now without nose.   OM OM OM
I walk now without feet.   OM OM OM
I grasp now without hands.   OM OM OM
I know now without mind.   OM OM OM
I am pure Consciousness.   OM OM OM
I am the womb for everything.   OM OM OM
I am the root for this world.   OM OM OM
I am the support for everything.   OM OM OM
I am the supreme abode.   OM OM OM
I am the centre.   OM OM OM
I am the foundation.   OM OM OM
I am the origin.   OM OM OM
I am the place of dissolution.   OM OM OM
I am Agadha Brahman.   OM OM OM
I am Aprameya Brahman.   OM OM OM
I am Aparichhinna (illimitable) Brahman.   OM OM OM
I am Avyapadesha (indescribable) Brahman.   OM OM OM
I am verily that Brahman which is
    indicated by the "Neti-Neti" doctrine and
    Bhaga-Tyaga-Lakshana of Vedanta.
I am that Brahman that resides in the
    Daharakasa or Hridaya-Guha of beings.
I am that Brahman which aspirants
    try to reach by Tapas, Brahmacharya,
    Satyam, Dama and study of Srutis.   OM OM OM
I am full   OM OM OM
I am the endless one   OM OM OM
I am changeless and imperishable   OM OM OM
I am of the form of wisdom   OM OM OM
I am all alone   OM OM OM
I am devoid of attachment   OM OM OM
I am devoid of body   OM OM OM
I am actionless   OM OM OM
I am devoid of enjoyment   OM OM OM
I am devoid of the symbol of sex   OM OM OM
I am the Ancient One   OM OM OM
I am an embodiment of peace   OM OM OM

I am Hari	OM OM OM
I am Sadasiva	OM OM OM
I am untouched by the senses	OM OM OM
I am without form, without limit	OM OM OM
I am beyond space and time	OM OM OM
I am in everything	OM OM OM
I am the basis of the universe	OM OM OM
I am everywhere	OM OM OM
I am existence absolute	OM OM OM
I am knowledge absolute	OM OM OM
I am He, I am He,	OM OM OM
I am the absolute One,	OM OM OM
I am the entire whole	OM OM OM
I am the liberated one	OM OM OM
I am the passive witness	OM OM OM
I am the subtle	OM OM OM
I am the Imperishable	OM OM OM
I am devoid of limbs	OM OM OM
I am originless	OM OM OM
I am peerless.	OM OM OM

8. NIRGUNA MEDITATION

I am pure spirit	OM OM OM
I am pure Bliss	OM OM OM
I am Immortal	OM OM OM
I am Nameless, Formless	OM OM OM
I am ocean of Peace and Bliss	OM OM OM
I am infinity	OM OM OM
I am Light of lights	OM OM OM

9. ABSTRACT MEDITATION

Meditate on Peace, Santi
Meditate on Bliss, Ananda
Meditate on love, bliss
Meditate on goodness

Meditate on Existence
Meditate on Consciousness.
This is abstract meditation
This is formless, attributeless meditation.
This is Nirakara, Nirguna meditation.

10. NIRGUNA DHYANA

I am the Truth
I am the secondless
I am the illuminator of all things
I am Kutastha
I am pure consciousness
I am the only Essence full of Chit
I am the Essence of Vedanta
I am Chidakasa
I am stainless, immaculate
I am the unconditioned, the emancipated.

11. REALISE THE UNITY OF ALL SELVES

I am one with the Universe   OM OM OM
I am one with Brahman or the Absolute   OM OM OM
I am one with every being   OM OM OM
I am the Self-Immortal   OM OM OM
I am in tune with the Infinite   OM OM OM
I am one with friend and foe   OM OM OM

12. I AM

I am, I exist.
I am Existence, Knowledge, Bliss, Absolute,
I am; therefore, I think.
I am the Immortal Soul.
I am the all-pervading, infinite spirit.
I am Atma Samrat, Self-king.
I am the Emperor of the Kingdom of Self.
I am the non-dual, blissful essence,
I am absolutely free, perfect and independent,
I am the Governor and Master of the Universe.

I am the Indweller of all beings.
I am self-luminous, self-existent.
I am self-knowledge, self-delight.
I am That I am, I am That I am,
Sivoham, Sivoham, Sivoham, Soham,
Satchidanada Svaroopoham.

13. I AM ONE

I am one.
I am the only one.
I am alone.
I am secondless.
I am non-dual.
I am Advaita.
I am one without a second.

14. I AM THAT I AM

Soham Asmi
Aham Asmi
I am That I am
I am That
I am.

15. I AM NECTAR

I am the water of Immortality
I am nectar.
I am sweet Ambrosia.
I am bliss eternal.
I am unalloyed felicity.
I am infinite joy.
I am ocean of peace.
I am fountain of Happiness.

16. FORMULA FOR VEDANTIC MEDITATION

Aham Atma Gudakesa (Gita, 10th Chapter).
Aham Atma Nirakara Sarvavyapi Svabhavat
I am Atma, formless and all-pervading. (Avadhoota Gita).

Aham Brahma Asmi
(I am Brahman),
Aham Bhuma Sadasiva
(I am Sadasiva the Infinite or the Unconditioned),
Aham Brahma Asmi Sivoham Soham,
Satchidananda Svaroopoham,
Hamsa Soham, Soham Hamsa
·(He am I, I am He; I am He, He am I),
Aham Brahma Asmi, Brahmaivaham Asmi;
I am Brahman, Brahman am I,
Sivoham, Sivah Kevaloham;
I am Siva, I am Siva the secondless.

17. VEDANTIC AFFIRMATION

I am immortal, all-pervading Soul.
I am changless, deathless Atma.
I am ever free, free, free.
I am omnipotent and omniscient,
I am infinite, eternal, indivisible Brahman.
I am all-full, Self-contained Spirit.
I am self-luminous, self-existent Purusha.
I am ever peaceful, all-blissful over-Soul.
I am Sat-Chit-Ananda Svaroopa.

18. FORMULAE FOR NIRGUNA MEDITATION

I

I am the one, subtle, immortal Reality.
I am the witness of the three states.
I am without parts and secondless.
I am pure, of the nature of knowledge,
I am eternal, self-luminous.
I am stainless, motionless and endless.
I am deathless, birthless and limitless.
I am attributeless and actionless.
I am eternally free and imperishable.
I am destitute of old age and decay.

Chidananda Rupa Sivoham Sivoham
I am Siva of the form of Knowledge Bliss.

II

I am all-strength, power and beauty.
I am life eternal.
I am boundless, limitless, everlasting.
I am ever free, free, free.
I am life glorious, wonderful.
I am perfect, pure,
I am Infinite, Immortal.
I am all-courage.
I am embodiment of wisdom, peace and bliss.

19. WHO AM I?

Sit calmly and enquire 'who am I?'
This will solve all life's problems
This will give you freedom and Immortality.
This will destroy all pain and sorrow.
This body of flesh and bone am I not,
It is inert, perishable, with parts,
The senses, eye, ear, nose am I not,
They are finite products of elements.
The five vital airs am I not,
They are inert products of Rajas,
The doubting mind am I not,
It is also inert, finite and perishable.
Satchidananda Brahman am I,
Nitya Mukta Suddha Buddha Brahman am I,
Nirakara, Nirguna, Nirvisesha Brahman am I,
Akhanda Paripoorna, Vyapaka Brahman am I.
Swords and weapons cut me not,
Fire and atomic bombs burn me not,
Water and deluge wet me not
Cyclone and wind dry me not.
Vedas, Bible, Koran, Avesta have sung of me,
Rishis, Sages and Yogis meditate on me,
Fire, wind, carry out My commands,

Intellect, senses, sun, get light from Me.
Infinite eternal, immortal soul am I,
All blissful, self-contained Atman am I,
All-pervading, self-luminous Purusha am I,
Birthless, deathless, Timeless, Brahman am I,
Unaffected, actionless, silent witness am I,
Source of Vedas, womb, substratum of this world am I,
Inner Ruler, Indweller, Homogeneous Essence am I,
King of all Devas, Progenitor of Hiranyagarbha am I.

20. HOW FREE AM I !

O free, O gloriously free,
Am I in freedom from birth and death,
From pain, sorrow, Karma and nescience,
All that dragged me back is rent asunder.
How free am I,
How thoroughly free from cares and anxieties,
It is the grace of the Lord
I am purged now of all impurities,
I dwell in the abode of silence,
Nothing can disturb or distract me.
I have won, I have won,
The wave of bliss sweeps over me now,
The breath of freedom sweeps over me now,
Nityamukta Svaroopoham,
I am eternally free Rasa or essence.
No bending, no kneeling,
No 'good morning sir'
No 'Ji huzur sir',
No 'obedient servant'
No 'I beg to remain'
But I am Emperor of the three worlds,
Atma Samrat, Svarat, Sel-fking.
Suddhoham, Buddhoham, Niranjanoham
Samsara Maya Parivarjitoham
Pure, fully illumined, spotless
Free from the taints of Samsara am I.

21. I AM THE ALL

I

I give power to the Vitamins.
I am the stimulant in coffee and tea.
I am nutrition in food stuffs.
I am the intoxicant in liquors and opium.
I am the attraction in women,
Gold, dollars, notes and cheques,
I am the celestial manna in heaven.
I am the essence in Vaccine injections.
I am the healing agent in all 'Pathies'
I am the power in Atom Bombs.
I am the strength of all Ministers and Dictators
I am the power in non-violence and truthfulness
I am the nectar in Sahasrara.
I am sound, language, OM and Vedas.
I am the universe, elements and Devas.
I am the goal, centre and ideal.

II

I am the all, I am all in all.
There is nothing besides myself.
I am the soul of the Universe, Visva Atman.
I am the Self of all beings, Antaratma,
I am the warp and woof of all,
I alone really exist.
I am here; I am there.
I am now, I was, I will be for ever.
There is neither distance nor space in Me.
I am the ocean of existence.
This world is a mere bubble in me.
A drop fell from me
And it became the universe.
My effulgence shines in the form of Brahma,
Vishnu, Siva, Devi, Vyasa and other Rishis.
My essential nature is amazingly wonderful.

22. I AM NIRMALA BRAHMAN

I am the Satya-Jnana Ananta Brahman.
I am the Nishprapancha, Nissamsara Brahman
I am Nitya-Nishkala Brahman.
I am Akhanda-Paripoorna Brahman.
I am Sadananda Brahman.
I am Nirmala, Niranjana Brahman.
I am the Brahman without caste, creed.
I am the beginningless, endless Brahman.
I am the Brahman without differences.
I am the diseaseless, decayless Brahman.
I am the Brahman without "this", "that", "I", "He", "You",
I am Amala, Asanga, Nischala Brahman.

23. I AM VIJNANA GHANA BRAHMAN

I am Atyanta Achala Brahman.
I am Atyanta Sasvata Brahman.
I am Kevala Sanmatra Brahman.
I am Kevala Chinmatra Brahman.
I am Kevala Nadanta Brahman.
I am Sankalpa-vikalpa-rahita Brahman.
I am nameless, formless Brahman.
I am Vijnanaghana Brahman.
I am Vilakshana, Sarva-adhisthana Brahman.
I am Pariccheda-rahita Brahman.
I am Svayamjyoti Brahman.
I am Dvandva Ahambhava-rahita Brahman.
I am Duhkha Soka Rahita Brahman.

24. I AM SVATANTRA BRAHMAN

I am Chaitanyamatra Brahman.
I am Niramaya Brahman.
I am Niratisayananda Brahman.
I am Svatantra Brahman.
I am self-existent Brahman (Svayambhu).
I am Aparicchinna Brahman.
I am Avyaya Ananta Brahman.

I am Suddha Vijnana Vigraha Brahman.
I am Tat Pada Lakshya Brahman.
I am Twam Pada Lakshya Brahman.
I am Nirbhaya Brahman.
I am Akshara Brahman.

25. I AM OMKARA SVAROOPA

I am that Para Brahma Svaroopa,
Where there is neither ignorance nor knowledge,
Where there is neither honour nor dishonour.
Where there is neither support nor the supported.
Where there are no limiting adjuncts of body, mind, etc.
I am the Pure Chaitanya,
Where there is neither bondage nor liberation!
I am the Absolute which the pure mind meditates upon!
I am Omkara Svaroopa—of the essence of OM!

26. I AM NIRAVARANA BRAHMA SVAROOPA

I am Advaita Para Brahman Svaroopa,
Which is beyond the reach of mind and speech,
I am the pure Satchidananda Brahman,
Where there is neither Subha nor Asubha,
Where there is neither sky nor air,
Neither fire nor water,
I am the pure Brahma Svaroopa,
Where there are neither Sankalpa nor Vasanas,
Where there are neither Vikshepa nor Avarana,
I am Satya-jnana-ananda Svaroopa,
Which is Sakshi for the whole world.
I am Chinmatra Svaroopa,
Where there are neither senses nor mind,
Where there is neither Drishya,
Nor the Triputi of Seer, Sight and Seen.

27. I AM PARA BRAHMA SVAROOPA

I am Para Brahma Svaroopa (the absolute) without
special attributes;

I am the Essence which all the Vedantic
                                    scriptures investigate;
I am Anandaghana, embodiment of Bliss;
I am the fruit of Maha Mouna—the Great Silence;
I am the Svaroopa wherein there are neither dualities
                                    nor opposites;
I am that Para Brahman wherein there is neither
                                    pleasure nor pain;
I am the Absolute wherein there is neither darkness
                                    nor light;
I am the Pure Consciousness which cuts the knots
                                    of the heart !

28. I AM SATYA SVAROOPA

I am Satya Svaroopa.
I am Santa Svaroopa.
I am Suddha Sukshma Svaroopa.
I am Vijnana Svaroopa.
I am Nirvikara Svaroopa.
I am Akhanda Ekarasa Svaroopa.
I am Poorna Svaroopa.
I am Nivritti, Sannyasa Svaroopa.
I am Prajnana Ghana Svaroopa.
I am Nitya Chaitanya Svaroopa.
I am Nitya Tripti Svaroopa.
I am Mukti Svaroopa.
I am Santi Svaroopa.
I am Satchidananda Svaroopa.

29. 1 AM CHAITANYA SVAROOPA

I am the Truth, the only living Presence!
I am the Svaroopa-essence which is greater than
                                    the greatest!
I am the One Homogeneous Essence without distinctions!
I am Akhandaikarasa Svaroopa—One indivisible
                                    Homogeneous Essence!
I am the Absolute which is beyond the reach of the Srutis!

I am Brahma Svaroopa without motion!
I am That which transcends everything!
I am Chaitanya Svaroopa without the six modifications!

30. I AM CHINMATRA SVAROOPA

I am Brahma Svaroopa, without the five sheaths!
I am the Absolute Consciousness which is within that within!
I am Brahma Svaroopa, without time. space and cause!
I am Chinmatra Svaroopa, which is the essence of
                              Wisdom alone!
I am taintless Chinmaya Svaroopa, full of Consciousness;
                        where there is no ignorance.
I am Poorna Para Brahma Svaroopa which the .
                  Akhandakara Vritti is illuminating!
I am Pure Consciousness which has neither cause nor effect!

31. I AM SUKHA GHANA SVAROOPA

1 am the Brahman that moves the mind.
1 am the Absolute without this world of names and forms.
I am the Eternity where there is no time.
I am the pure Brahman where there is.
Neither egoism nor the formidable lust.
I am the Brahman which transcends Gunas,
Which is beyond Sat and Asat.
I am the ever-steady "Sukha Ghana Svaroopa."
I am the Svaroopa where there is
Neither coming nor going,
Neither waking nor dreaming,
Where there is no space to move about,
Where there is Supreme Peace for ever,
Which fills all space everywhere.

32. I AM ANANDA GHANA SVAROOPA

I am a Kevala Para Brahma Svaroopa,
Where there is neither two nor three,
Where there are neither parts nor divisions,
Where there is neither counting nor measuring;

I am Akhanda Chidakasa Ananda Ghana Svaroopa.
I am Nishkala, Nirdvandva Svaroopa.
I am Niramaya, Nishkriya Svaroopa.
I am Nirakara, Niravayava Svaroopa.

33. I AM MAYA-RAHITA BRAHMAN

I am Maya-rahita Brahman
I am Desa Kala Vastu Pariccheda Rahita Brahman
I am Svajateeya, Vijateeya, Svagatha Bheda
Rahita Brahman,
I am Vasana Sankalpa Rahita Brahman,
I am Brahman without Maya,
I am Brahman without country, time and object,
I am Brahman without intrinsic, extrinsic and genus
species differences,
I am Brahman without desires and thoughts.

34. I AM FORMLESS, ATTRIBUTELESS BRAHMAN

I am Nirakara, Nirguna, Nirvisesha Brahman,
I am Nirupadhika, Nishkala Brahman,
I am Nirvikara, Nirvikalpa Brahman,
I am Ajara, Amara, Avinashi Brahman,
I am Asanga, Akarta, Abhokta, Sakshi Brahman.
I am Niravayaya, Nirliptha Brahman,
I am Akhanda Paripoorna Brahman,
I am formless, attributeless special characteristicless
Brahman.
I am Brahman without limiting adjuncts and parts,
I am Brahman without change and imagination,
I am Brahman without decay and death,
I am Brahman without attachment, doership
and enjoyment.
I am Brahman without limbs and attachment,
I am indivisible and All-full Brahman.

35. I AM TRIGUNATITA BRAHMAN

I am Trigunatita Brahman.
I am Dvandvatita Brahman.
I am Nada Bindu Kalatita Brahman.
I am Bhavatita Brahman.
I am Kalatita Brahman.
I am Mayatita Brahman.
I am the Brahman beyond the three Gunas,
I am the Brahman beyond the pairs of opposites.
I am the Brahman beyond Nada, Bindu and Kala
I am the Brahman beyond imagination.
I am the Brahman beyond time.
I am the Brahman beyond Maya.

Chapter Four

DHYANA YOGA SUTRAS

1. DHARANA

1. Dharana is concentration.

2. It is fixing the mind on an external object or an internal point or an idea.

3. Concentration is fixing the mind; meditation is allowing one idea to flow continuously.

4. Be serene. Be cheerful. Be patient. Be regular in your practice. Observe celibacy. Reduce your wants and activities. Mix little. Observe Mouna. These are aids to concentration.

5. Concentrate on Trikuti or heart.

2. DHYANA

1. Dhyana is meditation.

2. When you practise concentration, meditation and Samadhi at a time, it is called Samyama.

3. Meditation is the key to unlock the door of Moksha.

4. Meditation bestows intuitive knowledge and eternal bliss.

5. Cultivate burning dispassion, burning aspiration or longing for God-realisation. You will have wonderful meditation.

6. Shun Siddhis or psychic powers. They are obstacles in the path of Yoga.

7. Too much sleep, lack of Brahmacharya, laziness, rising up of latent desires, company of worldly people, overwork, overeating are all obstacles in meditation.

8. Meditate on the form of the Lord. This is concrete meditation.

9. Meditate on His attributes. This is abstract meditation.

3. MEDITATION

1. Dharana or concentration matures in due course into Dhyana (meditation) and Samadhi (superconscious state).

2. Meditation is prolonged concentration. The process of meditation is like the pouring of oil from one vessel into another in a steady unbroken stream.

3. Meditation is an effort in the beginning. Later on it becomes habitual and gives bliss, joy and peace.

4. Only when you have practised preliminary stages of Sadhana such as Yama, Niyama, you will obtain the full benefit of meditation.

5. In the one-pointed state, there cannot be more than one idea. One idea can go only if another idea enters the mind.

6. However intellectual you may be, you cannot concentrate without the help of some image or symbol in the beginning.

7. Success in meditation is quick in those whose practice and meditation are intense.

8. Meditation is a positive, vital, dynamic process. It transforms man into divinity.

9. Through regular meditation you can build an impregnable and invulnerable fortress. Maya cannot assail you.

10. Meditation is the key to intuition.

11. Meditation is the key to unfold the divinity or Atman, hidden in all names and forms.

12. Meditation is the key to spiritual illumination.

13. Meditation is the only passport to the satisfaction of life.

14. Meditation is an antidote to death.

15. Meditation is a vital part of daily living. Therefore meditate, meditate daily.

16. Even a little meditation daily will raise you a little higher and a little nearer to God.

17. The mind is refined by devotion and meditation.

18. As gold purified in a crucible shines bright, so constant meditation on the Atman makes the mind pure and effulgent with spiritual lustre.

19. A purified mind can grasp anything. It can dive deep into the subtlest subject, and understand even transcendental things.

20. Meditation releases a great amount of spiritual power. By constant meditation on the Self, one attains liberation.

21. Meditate upon purity and other similar qualities associated with purity—qualities like simplicity, guilelessness, frankness, truthfulness, open-heartedness, innocence, goodness, etc.

22. Attune yourself with the Infinite by stilling the mind, by silencing the thoughts and emotions.

23. Mind is the biggest radio. It is the receiving set. Attune it with the Infinite. Enjoy the supreme bliss of the Supreme Soul.

24. Meditate. Root yourself in Divinity.

25. Shut down in meditation the conscious mind—that part of your mind which thinks of the external world, your body and its wants.

26. Meditation on Brahman is the highest form of religion.

27. You can realise Brahman when you have stillness or serenity of mind.

28. O Ram, meditate regularly in the early hours of the morning. Let the mind taste the bliss of the Self.

29. The meditative mood comes and goes. Restrain the senses. Be eternally vigilant.

30. Be regular in your meditation and become more positive.

31. Sit for meditation at fixed hours. Brahmamuhurta, noon, evening, (dusk, twilight) and night.

32. Your life and your meditation must become one.

33. In deep meditation there is the first divine thrill in the heart with joy and bliss.

34. When you enter into deep meditation, you will realise balance, composure, serenity, peace of mind, steadiness, fearlessness, highest dispassion.

35. Inner spiritual strength, perfect peace, knowledge and bliss are the fruits of meditation.

36. Meditate regularly. You will attain the goal, God-Realisation.

37. Meditate. Have a glimpse of That. All dualities, all sorrows, all pains will vanish in toto.

4. ENQUIRY AND MEDITATION

1. Enquiry into Brahman leads to the Supreme good of man. Brahman alone is to be enquired into. Do thou enquire into That. Verily That is Brahman. Thou art That.

2. Brahman cannot be realised without Vichara or enquiry. Enquiry consists in investigation into the problem: "Who am I? What is bondage? How has the Samsara come into existence? What is Moksha?"

3. Diseases like enemies besiege the citadel of health. Kill these enemies by the sword of meditation and Brahmavichara.

4. O Nectar's son! Stand up and proclaim: 'I am Immortal Atman'. The nectar of life Eternal is flowing. Hasten! Close your eyes, meditate and drink freely.

5. Do not rise from your seat even for one or two minutes, until the mind has completely withdrawn itself and gets fully merged in the Lord.

6. You want great strength. You can get this strength only from within by meditating on: "I am the Atman. I am pure, all-pervading, Immortal Soul."

7. Where are you now? Have you progressed any further in the spiritual path? Or are you stationary? Or are you retrogressing? Find this out at once and take suitable measures for your spiritual advancement. Be quick. Be on the alert.

8. Worldly thoughts alone cause the round of births. Purify your thoughts. Entertain lofty Divine thoughts. Have the one thought "I am immortal, all-pervading Soul." You will be freed from the wheel of births and deaths.

9. Stand as a witness of your thoughts. Do not identify with them. They will pass away soon. The mind will divide into two. One portion of the mind will be the witness. It will watch. It will remain quiet and undisturbed. The other part of the mind will remain as the object of study or observation.

10. You cannot have spiritual life if you have not learnt to look within or introspect.

11. Emancipation is the final fruit of meditation. It is the natural and eternal state of the Self. It has neither beginning nor end.

12. You should strive by every means to make your life better by ceaseless mental discipline and meditation. Only by spiritual illumination you can obtain deliverance from the wearisome round of birth after birth.

13. Nothing short of knowledge of Brahman or the Absolute can make you happy. Therefore, strive ceaseless meditation on the Innermost Self.

14. Constantly repeat day and night "I am Satchidananda Brahman; I am ever-pure, ever-perfect, all-powerful, all-pervading." Thought is all-important. What you think, you become.

15. Become silent and hear the whispers of God. What a strange power there is in silence! Silence is more eloquent than a silvery speech. Meditate and enjoy silence. Hail silence! The harbinger of peace. O Silence! Thou art Peace itself. Thou art Brahman. Adorations to Silence.

The Process of Supreme Communion

16. Meditation is a stepping-stone for entrance into the regions of spiritual bliss. Therefore, meditate regularly and constantly with a pure heart.

17. There is a condition of the mind which is quite independent of the external objects. This is termed as natural state or indifference. Meditation is this state.

18. There is no other means of knowing the Truth than one's own intuition. Vichara, enquiry of 'Who am I?' and meditation open the door of intuition,

19. There is no other means to obtain a hidden treasure except digging. Even so, there is no other means except meditation on Brahman, the Supreme Self, to attain the final beatitude.

20. Dhyana or meditation is a process by which one attains mastery over the senses. Dhyana is the fixity of mind on God, and then constantly dwelling on God to the exclusion of all other objects.

21. Meditation includes all those spiritual exercises which are best calculated to make the mind rest peacefully in Brahman or the Eternal.

22. Meditation tunes and harmonises the mind. Meditation keeps the mind in tune with the Infinite.

23. The early stages of meditation are found fraught with difficulties. The meditator loses interest after some time and stops his Sadhana. It is a terrible mistake. Plod on, friend! Seek the company of senior aspirants. Live with your preceptor now.

24. The practice of meditation should become habitual. You can achieve this through constant practice. There is no other way.

25. You will attain even now the Supreme Bliss of Moksha or freedom, if you practise constant meditation on Atman with a pure heart.

26. Solitude, austerity, self-control, patience, absence of jealousy and moderation in food are aids to meditation.

The Meditator and the Meditated Become One

27. The conscious mental repetition of the same concept is Dhyana or meditation. When this becomes perfect one will attain Samadhi, where the meditator and meditated become one.

28. A thirsting aspirant is ever vigilant. His thoughts day and night are always set on Brahman, the Eternal. He ever delights in meditation.

29. Meditation releases great amount of spiritual energy. This spiritual energy destroys all evil thoughts and sublimates the sex-energy.

30. Take a bath in the Jnana Ganga in the early morning through meditation. Clothe yourself in the garb of saintliness. Drink the cooling beverage of contentment. Then take the breakfast of peace with the spice of joy and the sauce of bliss.

31. Just as the river Ganges flows to the east, slopes to the east, inclines to the east, so also the Yogi who practises meditation flows to Samadhi, slopes to Samadhi and inclines to Samadhi.

32. If an aspirant meditates regularly for a fairly long period of time, he must surely develop higher states of awareness. If he does not develop this, there must be some error in Sadhana. He may not be meditating. He may be building castles in the air or enjoying good sleep or Tandra, a half-sleepy state.

33. Drink the tonic elixir of immortality by practising regular meditation in the morning. Mix the elixir with a generous proportion of bliss and peace by doing Kirtan for half an hour.

34. The mind finds no rest anywhere. There is no ultimate satisfaction of desires. The fire of desire burns your heart intensely. Cool this fire by the nectar of Atman obtained through meditation.

35. The meditator sometimes gets stuck up anywhere or even side-tracked. He will have to be very vigilant and ever watchful.

36. The mind becomes serene and attains peace by meditating on the unity of the Ultimate Reality.

37. Even if you practise Nirakara, Nirguna Dhyana, meditation on formless, attributeless Brahman, you can have meditation on your Ishta Devata or Saguna Brahman. The grace of the Lord is necessary for obtaining success in Nirguna meditation. The Saguna Brahman and the Nirguna Brahman are one.

38. The cause of birth and death and all sufferings is ignorance. Knowledge of Brahman or the Absolute brings it to an end. Therefore attain Brahma Jnana through meditation on Brahman.

39. There is no greater gain than the gain of Atman, the Inner Self. With a view to this gain, worship your own self. Meditate on this constantly.

40. Silence invigorates, energises and revivifies. Meditate and enter the silence. Merge in silence. Silence is Brahman.

5. LIGHT ON MEDITATION

What is Meditation?

1. Meditation is the uninterrupted flow of one idea of God.

2. Meditation is the royal road to everlasting peace and bliss immortal.

3. Meditation is the key to intuition.

Pre-Requisites for Meditation

4. You cannot practise meditation if your mind is full of desires, and if your mind is diverted by any external objects.

5. If your mind is unruly, uncontrolled, if your heart is full of resentment and turbulence, there will be no meditation for you.

6. He who has practised Yama-Niyama and Pratyahara will obtain the full benefit of meditation.

7. Meditation is not successful without discipline and devotion.

8. Concentration leads to meditation.

Useful Hints for Sure Success in Meditation

9. When Sattva is predominant, the mind is calm and serene. Meditation becomes calm and steady.

10. Meditation must be done with great faith and great interest. You will feel enriched and encouraged in the spiritual pursuit through regular meditation.

11. When you sit for meditation, take a resolve, "nothing shall shake or move me. I will not get up until I realise the Truth." This is the kind of determination, the faith in the ultimate achievement, which can bring the goal nearer to you.

12. Meditate on the nature of God, on His attributes viz. Omnipotence, Omniscience, Omnipresence, etc.

13. Meditate on that Brahman who is endless, fearless, timeless, spaceless, birthless and deathless, free from old age, supreme and self-luminous.

14. Meditate regularly.

15. Sit for meditation at fixed hours.

16. Meditation should form part of your daily routine.

Coveted Experiences in Meditation

17. In deep meditation there is divine thrill in the heart, with joy and bliss.

18. In deep meditation you merge in the innermost Self or Atman and attain the inner core of Divine Experience. The ego gets dissolved. The mind ceases functioning.

19. In meditation the whole mind is wholly absorbed in one thing or ideal to the exclusion of everything else. The activity of the senses is totally withdrawn by the very nature of the absorption of the mind.

20. Meditation leads to Samadhi or superconscious state.

Fruits of Meditation

21. Perfect peace, knowledge, serenity, steadiness, fearlessness, dispassion, Samadhi, insight, illumination are the fruits of meditation.

22. Meditation paves the way for perfection.

23. Meditation transforms man into divinity.

24. Meditation dissolves doubts.

The Vital Secret

25. Meditation opens the door of Moksha.

26. Meditation flows in a pure heart.

6. THE PROCESS OF MEDITATION

Method of Meditation

1. Meditation is a process by which there arises intuitive experience or spiritual Aparoksha (direct) Anubhava or experience.

2. Practise silent meditation. Attain spiritual development and Self-realisation.

3. Sit erect in a position of ease. Repeat OM, meditating on its meaning. Free the mind from all distracting thoughts and desires.

4. If your meditation is imperfect, examine your heart. There may be still undercurrent of Vasanas or desires, attachment and egoism. The senses may still be turbulent. Still there may be craving for sense-pleasures.

5. The practice of meditation is the great scientific method of knowledge.

Importance of Meditation

1. There is no knowledge without meditation. The Yogi churns his own soul. Truth becomes manifest.

2. Meditation is the most important aspect of religious life. Right meditation is very important. It is a process of canalising the mind to take the form of the object of meditation.

3. Meditation on Brahman bestows immortality. There is no other way to Immortality.

Goal of Meditation

1. The object of meditation is the realisation of the transcendental consciousness through intuition.

2. He who follows the path of meditation knows his Self as Divine and one with God.

3. Meditation brings you nearer to Truth than anything else.

4. Meditation is Dhyana. It leads to the summit of Samadhi or Superconscious state.

5. When the transcendence of the Gunas has taken place through the evolution of intuition, the meditation ceases.

6. After reaching the Goal, the Yogi does not meditate. There is no object to meditate upon, because everywhere he sees the all-pervasive Lord.

Benefits of Meditation

1. Even a little meditation saves you from fear of death.

2. Constant practice of meditation will bring tranquillity and peace within.

3. Meditation fills the mind with cheerful, powerful, Sattvic thoughts.

4. By sustained meditation on the form of the Lord, the devotee will acquire the deepest love for the Lord.

5. In meditation you get directly an abundant supply of Sattva from the Lord.

6. An aspirant who meditates regularly enjoys peace, tranquillity, joy and a feeling of independence.

7. Meditation is a great tonic and revitaliser. Have serene meditation in the calm hours of early dawn and quiet hours of evening twilight.

8. By practice of meditation all the lower desires vanish, all personal thoughts will cease. There is only desire to be one with the Lord.

Obstacles in Meditation

1. Thinking of the past and anxiety about the future is a hindrance in meditation.

2. Memory or recollection is a great obstacle in meditation.

3. Ignore psychic experience and keep the mind alert and fixed in the object of meditation.

4. Meditation must be deep, regular, more serious and continuous.

5. Through Vairagya and meditation the senses are weakened and the mind merges itself in the Supreme.

6. Be moderate in food. Dwell in solitude. Meditate, leave anger; abandon pride.

7. Yama, Niyama, Asana, Pranayama become preliminary to meditation.

Mind in Meditation

1. In meditation the mind is turned back upon itself. The mind stops all the thought-waves.

2. The moment the mind is restrained for the purpose of meditation, the impressions, the sensations of the past, constantly disturb the meditation.

3. When the spiritual vision is developed through Sattva and meditation you will be able to see the subtler existence, the Devatas and the Soul.

4. When you develop intuition through meditation, realisation of Atman takes place.

Self-Realisation by Meditation

1. Meditate on the innermost Self ceaselessly. The mind will be absorbed in Brahman. You will attain Self-realisation.

2. Slay the ego or the false self. Sit motionless and calm. Meditate and realise the Atman.

3. When you have made considerable progress in meditation, you lose the awareness of the process of meditation. You even cease to be aware of yourself, what remains is only the object of meditation. There is only awareness of pure consciousness.

4. Intuition merges the subject and object of knowledge together with the process of knowing into the supreme Brahman.

5. Learn to find eternal peace and everlasting bliss in meditation on the Atman or the Self Supreme.

6. He who practises meditation regularly and vigorously enters into Samadhi and attains a direct cognition of the all-full Jnana or Wisdom. He attains the supreme state of Jeevanmukti devoid of this illusory universe though existent for others.

7. Meditate in silence regularly. You will get inspiration, peace and spiritual strength. You will catch the glory of God and the splendour of Truth. You will feel the immanence of Truth.

Two Forms of Samadhi
Meaning of Samadhi

1. Samadhi is a state of full wisdom. It is union with the Absolute.

2. In Samadhi or the state where there are no limitations, there is nothing like the knower and the known. It is all a homogeneous experience.

3. In the state of Samadhi the mind merges with the Absolute or Brahman. Individuality melts. Everlasting Bliss is attained. The sage is free from pain, sorrow, fear and delusion.

4. Samadhi is all unity or Atman alone.

5. The state where there is absolute consciousness, where the mind does not seek or is at perfect rest, where the knower and the known have become one is Samadhi.

6. Through the annihilation of the modifications of the mind, you can attain Samadhi.

Savikalpa Samadhi

1. In Savikalpa Samadhi there is the consciousness, "I am meditating," "Brahman is the object of meditation."

2. In Savikalpa Samadhi, there is the consciousness of the knower, knowledge and the known.

3. In the case of Savikalpa Samadhi there is the consciousness of duality but it is superficial and only apparent.

4. Savikalpa Samadhi is a state of preparation. Nirvikalpa Samadhi is the goal.

Nirvikalpa Samadhi

1. When the mind ceases functioning, when all thoughts subside, when all consciousness of the body and the outer world is effaced from the mind, the individual soul merges in the supreme Soul. This is the Nirvikalpa Samadhi.

2. Abandon all Sankalpas and become a Nirvikalpa.

3. A man who is dreaming in his sleep experiences many sufferings, but when he wakes, feels no concern with any of them, even so, he who rests in Nirvikalpa Samadhi or Atman will be beyond all the effects of Prakriti.

4. In Nirvikalpa Samadhi no individual consciousness remains, as the individual consciousness is merged in the universal consciousness

5. In Nirvikalpa Samadhi there is the absolute absence of the triad of knower, knowledge and the known.

7. SAMADHI

1. Samadhi is direct knowledge of the Supreme Self. It is superconsciousness.

2. Successful deep meditation will ultimately lead you to Samadhi or the superconscious state.

3. Samadhi is not the abolition of personality. It is the completion of the personality.

4. Experience of fullness is called Samadhi. It is freedom from misery. It is Bliss Absolute.

5. During Samadhi there is no movement of Prana. There is neither inhalation nor exhalation.

6. Samadhi is where there is no birth, no death, no decay, no disease, no pain, no sorrow.

7. All names and forms vanish in deep meditation. There is consciousness of infinite space. This also disappears. There is a state of nothingness. Suddenly there dawns illumination, Nirvikalpa Samadhi.

8. Nirvikalpa Samadhi is the realisation of the highest value.

9. During Nirvikalpa Samadhi the Reality is intuited in all its wholeness. It is the experience of oneness with the Absolute.

10. In Samadhi you attain illumination. You have Brahmic Superconsciousness, in place of the still Jiva-consciousness.

11. In Nirvikalpa Samadhi there is no object. There is cessation of all mental modifications.

12. The Supreme being is actually realised by the Yogi at the highest stage of his spiritual experience or Nirvikalpa Samadhi.

13. When the Raja-Yogi attains Kaivalya, the Gunas (qualities) go back to their origin, namely, the Prakriti or Pradhan.

14. Buddhi or intellect, Ahamkara or egoism, Manas or mind, Indriyas or the elements, are only the Parinamas or the modifications of the threefold Gunas (qualities). These also merge into their original sources, one after another.

15. Purusha alone is the seer, or Drashta. The Gunas and their modifications are the Drishyam or the seen.

16. During Kaivalya or Independence, Chitta, egoism, and Buddhi get liberated.

17. During Kaivalya the Purusha is established in his own state of freedom.

18. When the Purusha attains Kaivalya, the Gunas and their modifications have no more purpose to serve the Purusha.

19. Na Aham, Na Tum, Daftar Gum: No "I", no "YOU", the office of Prakriti is closed now for the liberated Purusha.

20. Sensual pleasure is nothing when compared with the bliss of meditation and Samadhi.

21. In Sahaja Samadhi, the Soham Bhavana becomes automatic, continuous and natural.

22. In Nirvikalpa Samadhi, there is not even the Soham Bhavana, as there is no one to feel Soham.

23. The superconscious experience is Turiya or the fourth state. It is Nirvikalpa Samadhi or the state of perfect awareness of one's real Svaroopa of oneness with the Supreme Being.

24. Close the door of the intellect; shut the windows of the senses; retire into the chamber of the heart, and enjoy the sleepless sleep of Samadhi.

25. Samadhi is superconscious state.

26. Samadhi is union with God.

27. The state of Samadhi is all bliss.

28. The meditator loses his individuality and becomes identical with the Supreme Self.

29. The state of Samadhi is ineffable.

30. In Savikalpa Samadhi or Samprajnata Samadhi there is Triputi or the triad, the knower, knowledge and the known.

31. In Savikalpa Samadhi the Samskaras or impressions are not burnt.

32. In Nirvikalpa Samadhi all the impressions are totally burnt.

33. In Samprajnata Samadhi there is complete inhibition of the functions of the mind.

34. The Yogi attains Kaivalya or Absolute Independence, freedom, perfection now.

35. Samadhi is an awareness of Reality.

36. Samadhi is superconsciousness. It transcends duality of all kinds.

37. In Samadhi the triad, known, knowledge and knowable disappear.

38. In Samadhi there is neither 'I' nor 'you' neither 'he' nor 'she' neither 'here' nor 'there' 'neither 'this' nor 'that' neither 'above nor below'.

39. It is a state of fullness and eternal bliss, everlasting joy and perennial peace.

40. In Samadhi there is no consciousness of anything internal or external.

8. INTUITION

1. Inner realisation or illumination transcends all philosophy. It is one's own experience or spiritual Anubhava.

2. You can attain Atma Jnana or knowledge of the Self through intuition and intuition alone.

3. The immediate knowledge through intuition or spiritual Anubhava unites the individual soul with the Supreme Soul.

4. Sensing is false knowledge and intuition is right knowledge.

5. Intuitive knowledge alone is the highest knowledge. It is the imperishable, infinite knowledge of Truth.

6. Trust your intuition, which will never fail you.

7. Without developing intuition, the intellectual man remains imperfect.

8. Intellect has not got that power to get into the inner chamber of Truth.

9. Through intuition alone you can catch the vision of the Real or Brahman.

10. He who has intuition attains immortality.

11. Sell your cleverness and argument and buy intuition. You will rest peacefully. You will be blessed.

12. Vichara or enquiry opens the door of intuition.

13. Thought cannot reveal Truth or Absolute.

14. Without the philosophy of intuition, the philosophy of the West is bound to remain imperfect.

15. The scientific attempts to prove the Infinite are futile.

16. The only scientific method is intuitional.

17. The solution of the problem of religious philosophy and science is the development of intuition.

18. Real cultural advance is not along the intellectual side, but along the intuitional side.

19. Intuition or spiritual experience or Brahma Jnana is never produced, because we do not know any stage when it was not in existence.

20. Intuition is the only touch-stone of philosophy.

9. SAMADHI AND DIVINE EXPERIENCE

1. That blessed state in which the mystery of life is revealed, that serene, and blessed state in which the meditator enters into sleepless sleep, is Nirvikalpa Samadhi.

2. Samadhi is not a state of lethargy. It is intense awareness of the Reality, the highest intuition which reveals to the meditator things as they are in which eternal peace is experienced.

3. There is a general spiritual anaesthetic which is superior to chloroform, ether, etc. That is Nirvikalpa Samadhi or the Superconscious state of a Yogi.

4. There is an absolute experience in the state of Nirvikalpa Samadhi. Samadhi is not a state of idleness. It is awareness of the Reality. It is the highest intuition.

5. He who has attained Nirvikalpa Samadhi or Oneness with the Supreme can never be separated from Him.

6. The experience of fullness is called Samadhi. It transcends duality of all kinds and is undisturbed by the ego. It is free from worry. There is complete satisfaction. There is a feeling of having attained all that was to be attained.

7. The perfection or culmination of Dhyana (meditation) is Samadhi. In the state of Samadhi the meditator realises his identity with the Supreme Self.

8. Samadhi leaves a permanent mark on the aspirant who experiences it. He who has experienced Samadhi becomes wise and illumined.

9. Samadhi or Nirvana or God-vision is the birthright of every human being. It is not the monopoly of Sannyasins or ascetics alone.

10. The requisites for the attainment of Samadhi are steadiness of posture, purity of heart, abstraction of the senses and one-pointedness of the mind (Ekagrata).

11. Mere talk or discussion on Samadhi, any amount of mere study of Yoga scriptures cannot help you in the realisation of Samadhi. You will have to practise Yoga with

sincerity, earnestness and tenacity. Only crying "food" will not appease your hunger. You must sit down and take the food. Then alone your hunger will be appeased.

The Dawn of Light Divine

12. Absolute Ananda is the Supreme Reality. Rise step by step from the sensuous place of experience to the transcendental spiritual experience wherein all names and forms vanish, self-delight alone exists.

13. For him who sees the all-pervading, tranquil, secondless, blissful Atman there remains nothing to be attained or known. Know this perfect Atman and attain eternal satisfaction and perennial joy.

14. Even if you get a momentary glimpse of the Supreme, a new element enters your heart. The whole heart is revolutionised. The inner man is changed. A wave of Supreme Joy sweeps over you.

15. If you taste even once the sweetness of spiritual bliss in meditation, it will be irksome for you even to think of mundane objects.

16. He who has realised Brahman becomes silent. Discussions and argumentations exist so long as the realisation of the Infinite is not attained.

17. He who has experienced the blissful nature of Brahman or the Supreme Being does not suffer any trouble from fears either physical or mental.

18. The satisfaction that results from sense-objects is dependent and limited, whereas the satisfaction consequent on knowledge of Brahman is limitless and independent.

19. God-vision is a cosmic experience. It gives a new orientation to life, a new perspective of Reality. It is an experience as a whole. The Saint of Godvision beholds the world of expression of divine glory (Vibhuti).

20. God-vision leaves its lasting impression on the meditator's consciousness. God-vision is not seeing or

sensing in any form. It is of the nature of an illumination or direct Anubhava.

21. Turiya is the last door which opens into the temple of the unspeakable Bliss of Brahman.

22. The term "intuition" inadequately and imperfectly expresses the Supreme Realisation. It is Anubhava or Aparoksha Anubhuti.

23. You can really know Truth through intuition or personal experience (Anubhava, Aparoksha Anubhuti).

24. The luminosity of intuition of Aparoksha Anubhuti is self-luminosity. The luminosity of Sattva is reflected luminosity.

25. Intuition of Brahman removes all miseries, pains and sorrows and brings in its train unexcellable bliss. Therefore, attain intuition through purity and meditation.

26. The Bliss which results from union with Brahman or the Eternal is ineffable. You will have to realise it yourself.

27. The feelings and thoughts are the same though the languages are different. Even so, religious experience is the same though religions are different.

Chapter Five

QUESTIONS AND ANSWERS

1. EASY PATH TO CONCENTRATION

Q. What is the easiest way for concentration?

A. Japa of the Name of the Lord. And, a very important point to bear in mind in this connection is that perfect concentration is just not achieved in a day; you should never despair and give up your efforts. Be calm. Be patient. Do not worry yourself if the mind wanders. Be regular in your Japa; stick to the meditation hour. Slowly the mind will automatically turn God-ward. And, once it tastes the bliss of the Lord nothing will be able to shake it.

2. BENEFITS OF MEDITATION IN BRAHMAMUHURTA

Q. What are the advantages gained by a Sadhaka, by meditating in Brahmamuhurta?

A. In Brahmamuhurta the mind is calm and serene. It is free from worldly thoughts, worries and anxieties. The mind is like a blank sheet of paper and comparatively free from worldly Samskaras. It can be very easily moulded at this time before worldly distractions enter the mind. Further the atmosphere also is charged with more Sattva at this particular time. There is no bustle and much noise outside.

3. WORLDLY THOUGHTS AND MEDITATION

Q. When I sit for meditation, I am assailed by different thoughts. When will the agitation subside?

A. In a big city there is much bustle and sound at 8 p.m. At 9 p.m. there is not so much bustle and sound. At 10 p.m. it is still reduced and at 11 p.m. it is much less. At 1 a.m.

there is peace everywhere. Even so in the beginning of Yogic
practice there are countless Vrittis in the mind. There is much
agitation and tossing in the mind. Gradually the
thought-waves will subside. In the end all mental
modifications are controlled. The Yogi enjoys perfect peace.

4. ENTRY INTO SAMADHI

Q. How to enter into Samadhi quickly?

A. Cut off all connections with friends, relatives etc. Do
not write letters to anybody. Observe Akhanda Mouna (vow
of continued silence). Live alone. Walk alone. Take very
little but nutritious food, live on milk alone, if you can
afford! Plunge in deep meditation. Dive deep. Have constant
practice. You will be immersed in Samadhi. Be cautious. Use
your commonsense. Do not make violent struggle with the
mind. Relax. Allow the Divine thoughts to flow gently in the
mind.

5. LORD HARI AND THE OBJECT OF
CONCENTRATION

Q. How to do Dhyana of Hari?

A. Mentally fix your mind at His Lotus Feet. Then
rotate the mind on His silk cloth (Peetambar), Srivatsa,
Koustubha gem on His chest, bracelets on His arms, earrings,
crown on the head, then conch, discus, mace, lotus in the
hands and then come to His feet. Repeat the process again
and again.

Q. Where to concentrate the mind?

A. In the lotus of the heart (Anahata Chakra) or the
space between the two eyebrows (Trikuti) according to your
taste and predilection.

6. CONCENTRATION

Q. On what can one concentrate?

A. Concentrate on a concrete form in the beginning, on
the form of Lord Krishna with flute in hand or on the form of

Lord Vishnu with conch, discus, mace and lotus in the four hands respectively.

Q. One man told me to look constantly in a mirror on a point in the midspace between the two eyebrows in the reflection of my face. Can I do so?

A. You can. This is one way of concentration. But stick to one method, to Rama's picture only. You can spiritually grow when you concentrate on Divine forms and meditate on his qualities.

Q. Why do people concentrate on Saligram?

A. It has got a power to induce concentration easily.

Q. I am concentrating on Trikuti, on Om figure and sound. Am I right in my concentration ?

A. You are right. Associate the idea of purity, Sat, Chit, Ananda, perfection etc., with Om. Feel that you are all-pervading consciousness. This kind of Bhava is necessary.

Q. What should I do to have deep concentration of mind?

A. Develop intense mental Vairagya. Increase the time of practice. Sit alone. Do not mix much with undesirable persons. Observe Mouna for three hours. Take milk and fruits at night. You will have deep concentration of mind. I assure you.

Q. The disciple needs words of encouragement. Often he wants to be in touch with his Guru. That is why I disturb you always. May I enquire now how the power of concentration increases.

A. You can write to me often. Disturbance concerns with the mind. There is always peace for one who lives in the Atman which transcends mind. Disturbances, troubles and afflictions can hardly touch such a person, who lives in the Spirit. Concentration increases by curtailing your wants and desires, by observing Mouna (keeping silence) for two hours daily, by remaining in seclusion in a quiet room for one or two hours daily, by practising Pranayama, by prayer, by increasing the number of sittings in meditation in the evening and at night, by Vichara, etc.

Q. Can Japa bring about concentration?

A. Yes. Do Manasika Japa.

Q. When I try to concentrate on the Trikuti, I get a slight headache. Is there any remedy?

A. Do not struggle with the mind. Do not make a violent effort when you concentrate. Relax all nerves, muscles and brain. Do gentle concentration in a natural manner. This will remove undue strain and consequent headache.

Q. The mind is still fickle in me and the flesh is weak. Attempts at concentration are sometimes successful, but often end in disappointment. The purification of mind is not easy. What do you suggest?

A. Your Vairagya is not pure. Develop Vairagya. Do intense Sadhana. Increase the period of meditation to 4 hours. Reduce your Vyavahara (activity). Go for seclusion for 3 months either to Rishikesh or Uttarkasi. Observe Mouna for full three months. You will have wonderful concentration and meditation.

Q. Why does the Yogi who does the Sakti Sanchar on his disciple ask him to give up all other kinds of Sadhana?

A. To develop intense faith, steadiness on the path and one-pointed or single minded devotion in one form of Yoga.

Q. I am doing Japa for two hours daily and Pranayama for half an hour. Can I have Ekagrata and Tanmayata in 2 or 3 years?

A. Yes, You can, if you are pure and sincere in your Sadhana.

7. MEDITATION

Q. What is Brahmamuhurta?

A. 4. a.m. in the morning is termed as Brahmamuhurta.

Q. Why is it eulogised by Rishis?

A. Because it is favourable for meditation on God or Brahman. Hence it is called Brahmamuhurta.

Q. What are the advantages gained by a Sadhaka by meditating at this particular hour?

A. At this particular hour the mind is very calm and serene. It is free from worldly thoughts, worries and anxieties. The mind is like a blank sheet of paper and comparatively free from worldly Samskaras.

It can be very easily moulded at this time before worldly distractions enter the mind. Further the atmosphere also is charged with more Sattva at this particular time. There is no bustle and much noise outside.

Q. Should I take bath before I start meditation?

A. If you are strong enough, if you are hale and healthy, if the weather and season can permit, if you are in the prime of youth, take a bath either in cold, lukewarm or hot water as desired. Otherwise wash your hands, feet and face with cold water. Do Achamana (sipping water with Mantra "Achyutaya Namaha Om, Anantaya Namaha Om, Govindaya Namaha Om").

Q. How to take to meditation or concentrate the mind (Ekagrata)?

A. First concentrate on the figure of Lord Hari with four hands for one year. Then take to abstract meditation on an idea. You can meditate on these: "Om Ekam, Akhanda, Chidakasa, Sarva Bhuta, Antaratma"—"One, indivisible Atman, the Indweller of all creatures, all-pervading, subtle consciousness like ether."

Q. My greatest difficulty is about concentration of the mind. The mind almost always is running away during my meditation. What is the remedy?

A. Strengthen your Vairagya and Abhyasa. Again and again you will have to bring the mind to the Lakshya. If you can make it run 50 times instead of 55 times, that is a great achievement for you. Mouna (vow of silence) will help you a lot in winter: You have your sittings in meditation in the morning, afternoon, evening and at night.

Q. What can I do besides Pranayama to elevate the mind when it gets dull, during meditation? May I use counter suggestions?

A. Whenever the mind gets dull, assert: "I am Atman, I am full of knowledge. I am Jnana Svaroopa. I am omnipotent—OM OM OM". The mind will be elevated and fixed in your meditation.

Q. A Yogi told me that while, meditating on God, he can hear the sound of Sri Krishna's flute and the Shankha Nada. Is it true? If so, how to hear it?

A. It is quite true. Concentrate upon Krishna's picture. You will hear those two kinds of sound. Close the ears with the two thumbs or a ball of yellow bees-wax beaten with cotton and concentrate deeply on the sounds you hear from the right ear. You will hear those sounds. Practise this at night.

Q. I would pray to you to give me some more instructions, some methods of Dhyana and some hints for getting along the right path.

A. Visualise every part of Sri Krishna's body with His ornaments, silk Peetambar, flute, etc., with closed eyes and keep the image steady. If the mind runs, if you cannot bring it back to the point, allow it to roam about for a while. It will settle down by itself after some wild jumping hither and thither.

Q. Why should we devote time for meditation? God is not desirous of our prayers.

A. The goal of life is Self-realisation or God-consciousness. All our miseries, birth, old age and death, can end only by realisation of God. Realisation can be had through meditation on God. There is no other way, my dear Ram. Therefore one should practise meditation. God prompts us to do prayers, Japa, etc., because, He is the Preraka (He who inspires our minds).

Q. Can I get help from God during meditation?

A. Yes. The indwelling presence that shines in your heart is awaiting with outstretched hands to embrace the sincere devotees.

Q. Is it advisable to do meditation after meal at night? A Grihastha is so much disturbed in the evening that he scarcely gets time to meditate.

A. Meditation at night, a second sitting, is absolutely necessary. If you have no sufficient time at night, you can meditate even for a few minutes say 10 or 15 before going to bed. By so doing the spiritual Samskaras will increase. The spiritual Samskaras are valuable assets or priceless treasures for you. Further you will have no bad dreams at night. The divine thought will be carried during sleep. The good impressions will be there.

Q. What is the difference between Japa and meditation?

A. Japa is the silent repetition of the name of the Lord. Meditation is constant flow of one idea of God. When you repeat Om Namo Narayanaya it is Japa of Vishnu Mantra. You think of conch, discus, mace and lotus flower in the hands of Vishnu, His ear rings, crown on His head, His Yellow silken Peetambar, etc., it is meditation. When you think of the attributes of God such as Omniscience, Omnipotence, etc., it is also meditation.

Q. Give me practical instructions on how to meditate?

A. Sit on Padma or Siddha Asana in a solitary room, keep the head, neck and trunk in one straight line. Close your eyes. Imagine that a big, effulgent sun is shining in the chambers of your heart. Place the picture of Lord Vishnu in the centre of a lotus flower. Locate the picture now in the centre of the blazing sun. Repeat His Mantra "Om Namo Narayanaya" mentally and see His image in your heart mentally from foot to head, His weapons in the hands, etc. Shut off all other worldly ideas.

Q. When I meditate, my head becomes heavy. How to remove this?

A. Apply Amalaka oil to the head and take cold bath. Dash some cold water on the head before you sit for meditation. You will be all right. Do not wrestle with the mind.

Q. Is seclusion necessary?

A. Absolutely necessary. It is an indispensable requisite.

Q. How long should I remain in seclusion?

A. For full three years.

Q. Can you suggest to me some solitary place for meditation?

A. Rishikesh, Hardwar, Nasik, Uttarkasi, Badri Narayan, Kankhal near Hardwar, Brindawan, Mathura, Ayodhya or Kashmir.

Q How shall I prepare myself for a contemplative life?

A. Divide your property between your three sons. Keep something for yourself to keep the life going. Distribute a portion in charity. Build a Kutir in Rishikesh and live there. Do not write letters to your sons. Do not enter into the plains. Then start meditation. Your mind will rest in peace now. Do this at once. You must hurry up.

Q. When I was living in Uttarkasi I had good Nishtha, exalted Vrittis and good Dharana. I have lost them now when I entered the plains even though I do Sadhana. Why? How to raise myself as before?

A. Contact with the worldly-minded people at once affects the mind. Vikshepa comes in. Mind imitates. Bad, luxurious habits are developed. Bad environments and bad association play a tremendous part and produce bad influence in the mind of Sadhakas. Old Samskaras are revived. I will ask you to run at once to Uttarkasi back again. Do not delay even a single minute. As the mind is formed out of the subtlest part of the food, it gets attached to that man from whom it receives its food. Do not be under obligation to anybody. Lead an independent life. Rely on your own self.

Q. Why do I not get success in meditation even though I am practising it for the last six years?

A. You have no Chitta Shuddhi.

Q. How can I find out that I have got Chitta Suddhi or not?

A. Sexual thoughts, worldly desires, unholy ideas, sexual Vasanas, anger, vanity, hypocrisy, egoism, greed, jealousy, etc. will not arise in your mind if you have Chitta Suddhi. You will have no attraction for sensual objects. You will have sustained and lasting Vairagya. Even in dreams you will not entertain evil thoughts. You will possess all virtuous divine qualities such as mercy, cosmic love, forgiveness, harmony and balance of mind. These are the signs to indicate that you have attained Chitta Suddhi

Q. How long will it take for a man to have Chitta Suddhi?

A. It depends upon the state of evolution of the man and the degree of Sadhana. He can have purity of mind within six months if he is a first class type of student. If he is a mediocre student it may take for him six years.

8. SAMADHI

Q. What is Samadhi?

A. It is oneness with God or Brahman.

Q. What kind of Samadhi did Tukaram, Ramdas, Tulasidas and other Bhaktas have?

A. Savikalpa Samadhi.

Q. Can there be any Vasanas in those who have attained Savikalpa Samadhi?

A. No.

Q. Describe their state?

A. These Bhaktas who had realisation had oneness with Ishvara, but they kept up their individuality also through a thin veil. They had all Divine Aisvarya. They were absolutely free from all sorts of worldly miseries. They were enjoying Divine bliss. They operated with their subtle Karana Sarira (causal body)

Q. What is Nirvikalpa Samadhi?

A. It is the superconscious state wherein the Jivatma dwells in oneness with Brahman.

Q. What is Maha Samadhi ?

A. It is the same as the Nirvikalpa Samadhi.

Q. What is Turiya?

A. It is the state of Samadhi wherein one rests in his own Svaroopa or Brahman. It is superconscious state wherein one acquires knowledge of Brahman. It is the fourth dimension according to a Russian Philosopher.

Q. How it is obtained?

A. Through Vichara, Vasana Kshaya or Manonasa (annihilation of mind).

Q. How to enter Samadhi quickly?

A. If you want to enter Samadhi quickly, cut off all connections with friends, relatives, etc. Do not write letters to anybody. Observe Akhanda Mouna (vow of continued silence) for one month. Live alone. Walk alone. Take very little but nutritious food, live on milk alone if you can afford. Plunge in deep meditation. Dive deep. Have constant practice. You will be immersed in Samadhi. Be cautious. Use your commonsense. Do not make violent struggle with the mind. Relax. Allow the divine thoughts to flow gently in the mind.

Q. Is it really possible to enter into Nirvikalpa Samadhi and be free from worldly affairs at that stage?

A. It is quite possible. If you can meditate for 6 hours daily you will get Nirvikalpa Samadhi. Introspect and see that you are free from all sorts of subtle varieties of pride, greed, lust, Moha and other attachments.

Q. Do you know any Yogi who can remain in Samadhi for some months by the practice of Pranayama?

A. I do not know.

9. EXPERIENCE IN MANTRA SADHANA

Q. What are the signs that indicate that the Mantra is really benefiting the Sadhaka?

A. The Sadhaka who practises Mantra-Yoga will feel the Presence of the Lord at all times. He will feel the Divine Ecstasy and holy thrill in the heart. He will possess all Divine qualities. He will have a pure mind and a pure heart. He will feel horripilation. He will shed tears of Prema. He will have holy communion with the Lord. .

10. THE METHOD OF INTUITION

Q. Is it proper to trust the method of intuition for the purpose of gaining philosophical knowledge? .

A. The phrase "method of intuition" is misleading as it may give rise to the opinion that intuition is only one among several methods of right knowledge. Intuition is the only method of non-relational external experience through which absolutely valid knowledge does not go beyond the intellect or reason, and hence they are inferior to intuition. Logical knowledge appears to be supreme as long as intuition is not gained. Even in the West where practical demonstrable knowledge alone is counted, the clock has come a full round and more and more philosophers are becoming alive to the importance of intuition and a correct appraisement of the part it plays in enabling man to obtain real knowledge.

11. SAHAJA SAMADHI AND NIRVIKALPA SAMADHI

Questions:

1. What is Sahaja Samadhi and what is its relationship or connection with Nirvikalpa Samadhi?

2. What part does the Breath, Soham, play in Sahaja Samadhi? Does the world exist in Sahaja Samadhi?

3. God men like Sri Ramakrishna said that man lives only 21 days after entering into Nirvikalpa Samadhi?

4. Why struggle for Nirvikalpa State, when one is happy and contented in Sahaja Samadhi?

Answers:

Sahaja Samadhi is, so to say, an "extension" of Samadhi so that it covers all the twentyfour hours of the day and not only when one sits in meditation. The Reality of God and the unreality of names and forms and the inner realisation that the individual self is none other than the Supreme Self that pervades everywhere and everything comes to stay in Sahaja Samadhi. The Samadhi that the Sadhaka strives to experience through Bahiranga and then Antaranga Sadhana comes to stay, in other words, becomes natural (Sahaja). The ego, the world, and one's own body appear like a glass-pane on which has settled a thin coating of moisture; you are able to see through it; yet you see the glass-pane itself on account of its moisture; the glasspane is transparent except for a slight opacity. The Yogi in Sahaja Samadhi perceives the world in exactly the same manner as a man who knows that a mirage is a mirage, admires one when he sees it, he sees the water-like spectacle without being deluded into believing it is actually water.

There is a slight Sattvic trace of ego in the Yogi who enjoys Sahaja Samadhi, which enables him to live to experience and to work. But, as he is rooted in the consciousness of SOHAM, he is not affected by living, by experiencing and by working. Lord Krishna has given the exact description of this state in the second Chapter (Sthita Prajna description).

12. STATES OF SPIRITUAL EXPERIENCES— THE AROMA OF SAHAJA AVASTHA

No one need struggle to pass from Sahaja to Nirvikalpa Samadhi; it is an automatic process. Even the struggle that the Yogi puts forth (if it may be called struggle) is intended only to maintain the Sahaja Avastha. The slender thread of Sattvic ego should be prevented from assuming Rajasic proportions. Though such downfall is very rare, we do come across such instances in our scriptures where a slight heedlessness spoils the game. If, as Lord Krishna puts it in the Gita, the Sahaja Avastha is maintained till the very end of life (till the Prarabdha is exhausted), one attains Brahma-Nirvana or Nirvikalpa Samadhi.

Sahaja being a God-conscious state, the Yogi vigorously engages himself in Lokasangraham. In selfless service and cosmic love, Karma is rapidly worn out, and the Supreme Culmination is hastened—at the same time all chances of even the slightest descent from the high Sahaja Avastha are prevented.

13. EXPERIENCES IN SAMADHI

Q. What are the experiences in Samadhi?

A. Experiences in Samadhi are beyond description. Words are imperfect. Language is imperfect. Just as the man who has eaten sugar candy cannot describe its taste to others, so also the Yogi cannot express his experience to others. Samadhi is an experience that can be felt intuitively by the Yogi. In Samadhi, the Yogi experiences Infinite Bliss and attains Supreme knowledge.

Q. Step by step what do we see or experience in Samadhi?

A. Steps in Samadhi differ according to the kind of Yoga. A Bhakta gets Bhava Samadhi and Maha Bhava Samadhi through purified mind and devotion. Sraddha, Bhakti, Nishta, Ruchi, Rati, Stayibhav, and Mahabhava (Premamaya) are the stages through which a devotee passes. A Raja Yogi gets Savichara, Nirvichara, Savitarka, Nirvitarka, Sasmita, Sananda and then Asamprajnata Samadhi through suppression of thoughts and Samyama. He gets Rithambara, Prajna, Madhubhumika, Dharmamegha and Prasankhya, etc. A Jnani or Vedanti experiences ecstasy, insight, intuition, revelation, illumination and Paramananda. He passes through the stages of Moha, darkness, void, stage of infinite space, stage wherein there is neither perception nor non-perception, stage of infinite consciousness and bliss. Subhechha, Suvichara, Tanumanasi, Sattvapatti Asamsakti, Padarthabhavana, Turiya are the seven stages through which the Vedanti passes. A Jnaniyogi is always in Samadhi. There is no "in Samadhi" or "out of Samadhi" for him.

14. CONTEMPLATION AND SUPERCONSCIOUS EXPERIENCE

Q. What is the difference between contemplation and meditation?

A. Contemplation is Manana or reflection on what one has heard. Meditation is to keep one idea of God or Brahman on the mind. Contemplation results in meditation. Meditation results in Samadhi.

Q. Can one in Nirvikalpa Samadhi break it at will?

A. Yes.

Q. Whether a man in Samadhi cannot be misunderstood by outsiders as dead and lost?

A. A Yogi in Nirvikalpa Samadhi will be misunderstood by outsiders as dead and lost.

Q. Is there any difference between meditation and worship?

A. Offering of flowers, waving of camphor (Arati), reciting hymns, etc., constitute worship. Meditation is the keeping up of a continuous flow of one idea of God or Atman.

15. EXPERIENCES AND MYSTICS

Q. Some aspirants say they see lights and hear Anahata sounds during meditation. Are these all correct?

A. These are all the signs of the first stage in concentration. They are correct.

Q. Can you describe the state of Nirvikalpa Samadhi?

A. It is indescribable. It is the state of one's own spiritual experience. There are no words to describe it. It is an experience of supreme peace and bliss. Can anyone describe the state of sugar-candy or apple?

Q. Then how to attain this final Samadhi?

A. Purify your heart. Meditate. You will attain Samadhi.

Q. How can we know that the experience that mystics or saints describe is true?

A. There is a Power in their words. Their contact is elevating and inspiring. They are ever peaceful, joyful, blissful. They are free from lust, greed, anger, likes and dislikes. Their experiences tally with the experiences of sages described in the Gita and the Upanishads.

16. INTUITION AS EYE OF WISDOM

Q. Once again I refer to the thought force and your experiences about it. Will you show that to me?

A. Please sit down with a concentrated mind. You will experience the thought transference. Close your eyes.

Q. How would you define Intuition?

A. Intuition is spiritual Anubhava or experience. It is the divine eye of wisdom.

Q. Suppose I wish to pay Rs. 100/ to somebody, but I am poor. The heart cries to pay but the reason declines.

A. This is not intuition.

Q. Do you believe that actions done with intuition are always right and correct?

A. Yes. They are infallible, because the Yogi is in contact with the Divine or Supreme wisdom.

APPENDIX

100 SELECTED APHORISMS FOR MEDITATION

1. Wisdom can dawn only in a pure and steady mind. Therefore purify your mind and be still.

2. The main obstacles to meditation are sleepiness, lust, fickleness and day-dreaming.

3. God is beyond the realm of gross thought but a pure, subtle and concentrated mind can realise Him in meditation.

4. The lives of saints are compasses on the way to liberation.

5. Bitter pills have blessed effect.

6. The practice, which consists of meditation on the Omnipresent God, remains the easiest, shortest and surest way to get God-Realisation.

7. The salt of life is selfless service. The bread of life is all embracing love. The water of life is purity.

8. The sweetness of life lies in devoted surrender. The perfume of life is generosity, its support is meditation and Self-realisation its goal.

9. The fruits of meditation are inner spiritual strength, perfect peace, realisation and bliss.

10. The man who becomes a victim to lust and anger is inferior to animals.

11. Wrath is the daughter of ignorance, the sister of jealousy and the mother of hard-heartedness.

12. Without surrender to the Lord, our life is empty. Without surrender you live in vain.

13. Surrender is important. It is a great force. It is the stream of life.

14. Self-surrender liberates. It destroys pain and gives peace.

15. Spiritual growth is gradual. It is a step by step development. Therefore do not try in great haste to do all sorts of Yogic, heroic deeds, or strive for perfection within 2 of 3 months.

16. Step by step, you must climb the ladder of Yoga. Step by step you will have to advance on the spiritual path.

17. There is a mysterious power in prayer. Prayer can work wonders.

18. Prayer can move mountains. But it must be intense and it must come from the heart.

19. You are not the perishable body. Your being is of the substance of Atman. Identify yourself with Atman.

20. The way which leads to saintliness is regular meditation. The foundation of saintliness is self-control (Yama) and Niyama.

21. All-embracing love is the light of saintliness. Its robe is virtue, and to esteem all things alike is its sign.

22. No light of this world can be compared with Self-realisation or the vision of God (Brahman).

23. There is no greater treasure than contentment.

24. There is no greater virtue than truthfulness.

25. There is no greater bliss than that of the Soul.

26. There is no better friend than the Atman.

27. Eat a little. Breathe deeply. Speak with kindness. Work with energy.

28. Think useful thoughts. Remain faithful to your resolutions. Be earnest, steadfast and quick at your job. Be courteous. Pray whole-heartedly.

29. Be courageous in endurance. Bear patiently. Concentrate with highest alertness. Meditate earnestly and realise fast.

30. Sensuous pleasures are nothing compared with the bliss of meditation and highest consciousness.

31. Close the doors of the intellect, shut the windows of the senses, withdraw into the still chamber of your heart and enjoy the sleepless sleep of highest consciousness.

32. Without the control of the senses and the thoughts, spiritual growth is not possible.

33. Abuse and criticism is nothing but a play of words, mere vibrations in the air.

34. Rise above any praise and identify yourself with the highest existence.

35. Meditation induces a fullness of spiritual power, in most peace and life energy.

36. Through prayer and meditation, continence and non-violence, human nature is purified.

37. The fruits of meditation are inner power, unalloyed peace, realisation and bliss.

38. Every set-back increases your power to rise to a higher rung in the ladder of Yoga.

39. Ignorance begets unhappiness, moodiness and destruction. Become Self-realised and be in harmony with all.

40. Every obstacle is your opportunity to develop will-power.

41. Be patient in troubles, dangers and grief; be hard like a diamond and overcome the obstacles.

42. Lust destroys life, lustre, personality, the life-force, memory power and reputation, holiness, peace, knowledge and devotion. Therefore kill lust.

43. Inexperienced students mistake their own imagination and impulses for the inner voice.

44. The secret of renunciation consists of renouncing egoism and lust.

45. Live in the world, but be not worldly-minded. He who lives in the world and reaches perfection in the midst of all temptations is the real hero.

46. God will never forget you, even if you forget Him through the power of ignorance.

47. Do not mix with evil company.

48. Within you is an immeasurable, inexhaustible spring of knowledge and power. Learn to draw from this well. Delve deep into yourself, and dive into the holy waters of immortality.

49. Learn to understand the laws of the universe and move in tune with the world.

50. Every obstacle gives you opportunity to develop strong will and to grow in strength.

51. Grow. Expand yourself. Develop all positive and good qualities, Daivi Sampat, like: large-heartedness, commonsense and courage. Step on the spiritual path and recognise: I am the immortal Self.

52. Do not go against the laws of nature.

53. Comfort and console the unhappy.

54. Shun diplomacy and hypocrisy.

55. Destroy your pleasure-centres.

56. Feel oneness with all.

57. Raise your mind by spiritual thoughts, expand it by intensive one-pointed thoughts of Brahman.

58. Every work is a sacrifice to the Lord. Feel that all beings are His images (creation).

59. See God everywhere, in every face.

60. God pervades the whole universe. He wears the robe of a beggar. He aches in pain under the mask of the sick. He wanders in rags through the forests. Open your eyes. See Him in everybody. Serve all. Love all.

61. Three things you should acquire: Trust in God, atonement and readiness to sacrifice.

62. Three things are admirable: Truthfulness, honesty and large-heartedness.

63. Three things are to be controlled: Tongue, anger and restless thoughts.

64. Three things are to be cultivated: Cosmic love, kindness and patience.

65. Three things are loveable: The wish for liberation, the company of saints and selfless service.

66. Three things are to be avoided: Covetousness, brutality and triviality.

67. Three things are to be renounced: Lust, evil company and fruits of actions.

68. Three things combine into one synthesis: The Yoga of service, of surrender, and of knowledge.

69. To be childlike, is good. But to be childish, is not good.

70. To be devotional, is good. To be emotional, is not good.

71. To have strong will-power, is good. To be stubborn, is not good.

72. To hold fast to one ideal, is good. To be intolerant, is not good.

73. To be courageous, is good. To expose oneself to danger is not good.

74. To be straightforward, is good. To expose other's fault, is not good.

75. Be kind, but firm and decisive; be gentle, but bold; be simple, but dignified.

76. The best way to get rid of some fault is to think ten minutes of the opposite virtue, and to practise the latter during the day.

77. Service is religion. Serve, Love, Give, Purify.

78. Be good, do good, be kind, be pure.

79. Listen, reflect, meditate, realise.

80. Trust at every step in the grace of God. Speak to the Lord like a child. Open to Him your heart. His grace will immediately come to you.

81. Avoid unnecessary talk.

82. Gentle words break no bones, but they break the hard heart.

83. There is but one caste, the caste of mankind.

84. First of all find peace within yourself through discipline and meditation, then go and propagate peace to the world.

85. Adapt, adjust, accommodate. Bear insult and injury.

86. Pray for him who tries to harm you, and persecute you.

87. Serve him who speaks ill of you.

88. Love him who wants to do injustice.

89. What purifies the heart—that is virtue, what befouls the heart—that is sin.

90. That which brings you closer to God is virtue. That which thrusts you into the dark abyss of ignorance is sin.

91. Whatever gives you peace, joy, satisfaction and cheerfulness that widens the heart, that is virtue. What gives you restlessness, moodiness, depression, that is sin.

92. Insatiable is lust. It is the source of pain, grief, misery and unhappiness.

93. To be jealous is pitiable; to be selfish is shameful; to be compassionate is divine; to be patient and enduring is manly; to be without lust is profitable; and to be calm and relaxed is admirable.

94. Evil thoughts are just as evil as evil deeds.

95. Real Yoga is grasping of higher truth through conscious communion with God.

96. The more you run after sense-pleasures, the more restless and agitated you will be.

97. Be fully awake in all parts of your being. Be always alert and busy. Your presence should speak more than your words.

98. The spiritual practices should give you rich internal life, spiritual value of things, and the ability to remain calm under all circumstances.

99. Have a soft heart, a generous hand, a kind word, a balanced opinion, and an unprejudiced mind and lead a life of service.

100. You are never alone. God is always with you and
in your heart. He is very close to you. He desires you more
than you Him. Therefore drop all fright and fears.